The CAMP System

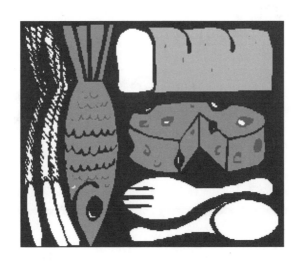

Learning to Live in Balance and Harmony with Food

Frederick Burggraf

The CAMP System: Learning to Live in Balance and Harmony with Food

First Edition: November 2000

ISBN 0-9706006-0-7

DayOne Publishing
P.O. Box 676
Charlotte Hall, MD 20622

www.MindfulEating.net
www.MindfulEating.org

Printed in the United States of America by EBSCO Media, Birmingham, Alabama.

The CAMP System

Table of Contents

Preface i

1. How to Use this Book 1
2. How the CAMP System Came to Be 4
3. Basics of the CAMP System 15
4. The CAMP Journal 19
   Practice: The Journal 26
5. Control 28
   Practice: Control 40
6. Attitudes 43
   Practice: Getting New Attitudes 55
7. Mindful Eating: Arriving 57
   Practice: Arriving at Food 65
8. Mindful Eating: Awakening 67
   Practice: A Simple Strategy 70
   Practice: The Raisin Encounter 72
   Practice: Awakening to Food 74
   Practice: Mindful Six-cracker Snack 76
   Practice: Eating and Reading 78
   Practice: Eating and Television 78
   Practice: Eating and Listening 79
   Practice: Eating and Speaking 79

9. Mindful Eating: Tuning In 82
        Practice: Finding Your HQ 84
        Practice: Tuning in to Eating 86
10. Mindful Eating: Service 90
        Practice: Mindful Food Shopping 91
        Practice: Mindful Soup 94
        Practice: Putting Away the Dishes 96
11. Portions: Challenges 98
        Practice: How Many Potato Chips? 103
        Practice: You're In Control 104
12. Portions: Sensation 107
        Practice: Popcorn Snack and Clearing 111
13. Portions: Boundaries 114
        Practice: Finding Your Bite Size 116
        Practice: The Cookie and Tea Encounter 119
        Practice: Cutting Up Food 122
        Practice: Pizza 123
        The Two Plate Strategy 124
        The Double Circle Strategy 127
        The Counter Strategy 128
        The CAMP Buddy Strategy 129
14. The Complete CAMP system 131
        Practice: A Basic CAMP Meal 133
        Practice: A CAMP Salad 135
        Practice: At the Buffet 138
        Practice: Fast Food 140
15. Balance and Harmony (Maintenance) 143
        Practice: Chocolate! 147
16. Frequently Asked Questions about the CAMP System 150

Preface

This book will teach you a new way to eat.

If you're a typical eater, you give very little thought to what you're eating and how you are eating it. You probably don't consider how big a bite you take each time or how fast you chew it. And it's likely that you never stop to contemplate the effort it took to bring that food to your table or plate. The CAMP system will open your eyes to these ideas, change the way you eat and help you to learn about your own relationship with food.

I am not a doctor, psychologist, psychiatrist, nutritionist or dietician. If I were, this book would have been similar to dozens and dozens of books already on the market. My background and perspective is that of an educator, a spiritual seeker and a very heavy overeater who found—finally—a system of weight management that made sense, that worked, and that actually made a lasting difference in my relationship with food and my attitudes about food.

This book is *not* medical advice, nor is it a book on the psychology of eating. If you're looking for such guidance, please look elsewhere. Just as people can be addicted to alcohol or nicotine or gambling, people can be addicted to food. If you suspect you have deep-seated problems and issues with food, I urge you to seek professional help. Food addiction and other serious eating disorders are far beyond the scope of this book.

This book will *not* talk about exercise. Exercising is a wonderful part of a healthful lifestyle and I highly recommend it, but if you're interested in such information, seek other sources. With or without exercising, the CAMP system can work wonders on bringing you back into balance and harmony with food.

This book is *not* a diet book; it will *not* talk about what foods you should and should not eat. If you're interested in diets, you can find many books on diets. Dieting did not work for me or for millions of others. If you have tried diets before and they didn't work in the long run, then this book is for you.

I *am* a firm believer that meals should have nutritional sanity behind them. But the CAMP system is not concerned with *what* you eat; rather the system centers on *how* you eat and *how much* you eat.

In fact, if you are currently on a diet that is not working, I recommend that you abandon it. Go back to eating normally, whatever that may mean. Get out of the diet mindset. If counting calories didn't work for you the last three times you tried it, it won't serve you any better this time. Begin on the CAMP system without the extra layer of the diet. Take a break; start from scratch. Be gentle with yourself and learn a new way of eating rather than potentially punishing yourself under the regimen of the diet.

The CAMP system is not a quick fix—don't expect to simply read this book and then watch the pounds melt away. The system requires effort, commitment, practice and persistence. It is a discipline that requires some rather hefty changes in your view of food and lots of practice.

But in its special way, the CAMP system is a minor miracle. If someone had told me a year ago that I could lose 60 pounds while eating the foods I love and doing very little exercise, I wouldn't have believed him. And yet that is exactly what the CAMP system did for me. Even more importantly, I now have a brand-new attitude about food, an enduring new relationship with food and I'm in control again. These are the real gifts of the CAMP system.

Acknowledgements

I would like to extend my thanks to the individuals who helped me with this book.

To the very first CAMP class members I extend a very special appreciation: they took a chance, believed in me and CAMP, and taught me far more than I taught them. Thanks to:

John Gladys	**Cyndi Otts**
Fred Hall	**David Pounds**
Julie Heath	**Dave Reed**
Judith Jenkins	**Beth Roth**
Jane Lancaster	**Janice Walthour**

To *all* the CAMP students and clients who came after the first group, I extend my deepest gratitude. The CAMP system continues to grow and mature through your interest and insights.

Thanks also to **Dr. Carol Marcy** for graciously hosting the first CAMP class at her Healing Center on Joy Lane, and for her continuing and untiring support of my program.

I extend heartfelt thanks to my editors: **Jeff Foster, Dr. Lois Knowles** and **Marianna Nystrom**, whose wonderful ideas and constructive criticisms brought sturdiness and elegance to my first wobbly manuscript.

And I give bushels of loving thanks to my wife **Karen**, who shared the CAMP journey with me and became the first CAMP convert.

Fred Burggraf
November, 2000

1.

How to Use This Book

When it comes to the topic of weight control, nearly everyone wants a quick fix. We buy diet pills and sit back and wait for them to work. We drink our liquid lunches with a hope that they will melt the pounds away forever. We spend much of our lives looking for the magic elixir, the secret potion, the no-effort solution to our weight woes.

The sad and inescapable truth is that no potion exists, the magic elixir is not to be found. To manage weight—and to manage it permanently—requires real effort, commitment and persistence.

The CAMP system is no different. Although the system itself is rather simple and non-mysterious, its power and effectiveness will depend completely on your level of effort. Its techniques and skills require practice, day in and day out. Over time, you should see improvements in your own performance with the system, and these improvements will be reflected on your bathroom scales or on your belt as well as in your life-long attitudes about food and yourself.

If you purchased a book on how to play the piano, you might be tempted to jump to the back of the book so you could get to the keyboard right away. Such a strategy, however, would be futile—by skipping all the chapters on practicing the piano, you would be terribly unprepared to understand the chapters near the end of the book. No one ever learned to play the piano for concert performance by jumping to the back of the book. In fact, no one every learned to play the piano simply by reading about it. One learns to play the piano by playing it, starting with the basics and building on them each day. Practice is the key.

The same is true with the book you're reading now. This is a book about *doing*. As you practice, the skills that seemed foreign or new will become second nature. So resist the temptation to jump to the back of the book. Instead, read it from the beginning. Do all of the suggestions and strategies as they appear. Take your time; don't try to rush the process. And don't skip any sections—you'll only shortchange yourself if you do.

Throughout many of the chapters there are "Practice" sections. These are activities that will help you learn the techniques, strategies and approaches of the CAMP system. I urge you to actually do these activities and integrate them into your life. Learning the CAMP system is like learning to ride a bike: you can read about it all you want, but until you actually get on the bike you won't get very far in applying the principles and mastering the skills you want to learn.

At the end of many of the chapters is a "Progress" section that summarizes what you should be doing at that point in the system. Starting with chapter 4, each chapter of this book introduces a new skill or activity. By working through the book sequentially and slowly, you'll gain the skills over time and at your own pace. When you feel you've got the main idea and skill from one chapter and you're ready for the next action of the CAMP system, move on.

Near the very end of this book is a chapter that answers frequently asked questions regarding the system. This chapter will summarize the system and many of the points made throughout the book. If you must "jump ahead," this chapter would be the best way to get an overview of the system.

The CAMP system works, but only when you put energy and commitment into it. For this reason, consider making a commitment to the system for 60 days. For the next two months, no matter where you are in your life, try all the suggestions and strategies and activities. At the end of 60 days, you'll be able to make a genuine assessment of how valuable the CAMP system is to you.

The CAMP system has worked its miracles for me and many others. If you apply your commitment and energy to it, it can work its miracles for you as well.

2.

How the CAMP System Came to Be

I was an unhappy fat man.

In 1992, at the age of 45, I had finally quit smoking after more than 27 years of puffing away. During the years after I quit, I went from a svelte 170 pounds (size 34 pants) to a ponderous 242 pounds (size 42 pants). And I found myself living as a very sad, obese person.

I had a number of health problems related to being overweight. One of the more serious was sleep apnea, a condition where my throat would close up during sleep, causing me to gasp for air many, many times each night. Usually, I'd wake up in the morning more tired than I was when I went to bed.

Then there was the fact that I couldn't eat a meal without sweating, often heavily. The large amount of food I ate was adding so much work to my already overloaded system that every meal was like hard labor.

I couldn't keep my shirts tucked in; my belt was forever slipping down. I felt like a fashion idiot, and my self-esteem suffered.

When I saw photographs of myself or a glimpse of my unexpected reflection in a store window, I would react with surprise and shock. "Who is that fat man there? That can't be me!" My mental image of myself as a skinny person never matched what I was seeing in the mirror or in a picture.

Of course, had I tried dieting many times, with all the calorie counting and liquid lunches and watching fat content and hating exercises. I avoided foods on a list longer than my pants were wide.

Did I lose weight? Yes.

Did I eventually gain it all back? Also, yes. My weight went up and down like a Death Valley thermometer and generally I was miserable. Like most people do, I found it too hard and too depressing to stay on a diet and so, eventually, I gave up and began eating like old times. The bathroom scales, an important tool during my diet days, got pushed out of sight. It was my theory that if I didn't know how much I weighed, then I was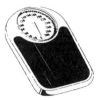

Welcome to enemy territory

safe—after all, it's only the weight you *know* about that matters!

The Moment of Truth

Then, in the spring of 1999, I developed sciatica, a severe condition of intense pain shooting down my legs whenever I stood or walked. I let it go for a few months, thinking it would get better. But it didn't—in fact, it got worse and worse. The time finally came to see a doctor.

I dreaded that moment, because I suspected that part of my doctor's exam would be (shudder) **getting on the scales**.

Sure enough, about a half an hour into the exam the dreaded moment came. On the scales I went and I watched as my doctor slid the metal counterweight across the bar. And kept sliding it. Still more. Finally, she stopped at 225. My heart sank. Although it wasn't my all-time high weight of 242, it was bad enough.

I knew what was ahead: a discussion with my doctor of why it's important to lose weight and some strategies for getting started. My doctor was wonderful in that she didn't set any immediate weight goals and that she understood fully the difficulties of losing weight.

But I knew that I couldn't diet again. I just hated it too much. What's worse, I knew that I couldn't count on exercising to help; my back was hurting too much. No, I had to try something very different, something life-changing, something at a deeper level than counting calories and food exchanges and fat percentages and spending hours on a treadmill.

Why Diets Didn't Work For Me

That visit to the doctor forced me to look at my dieting of the past. I wondered why diets had failed me. It made sense to me that if I could figure out why my diets hadn't worked, it just might make it easier to come up with something that would actually succeed.

After much thought, it occurred to me that my diets failed me for eight main reasons:

1. Diets deprived me of what I loved.
2. Because of the deprivation, my diets caused resentment.
3. Diets are systems ripe with the possibilities of shame and guilt.
4. My diets were, by their very nature, temporary.
5. My diets didn't train me to eat less.
6. My diets didn't change my attitudes about food.
7. Diets missed the point. They called attention to the food, when the real problem was something within me, something much deeper and more fundamental.
8. Diets take away control.

Let's explore each of these and see what they tell us.

1. Diets deprived me of what I loved.

I learned to eat fat and sugar and all that other "bad" stuff when I was a little kid. It wasn't my parents' fault; back in the late 1940s not much was known about foods and their long-term effects on health and fitness. So I developed a taste for all of the wonderfully depraved foods, and I learned that that's what good food tastes like.

This was fine until later in my life I had to face my first diet. The diet's message was hard to take: "I don't care what you learned to like—you can't eat that anymore. No more hamburgers. No more fried chicken. No more doughnuts, cheese, red meat, pink meat, blue meat, purple meat. Actually, you're allowed just three things: raw broccoli, unbuttered toast and water. And go easy on the toast and broccoli."

But wait a minute! All the foods I can't have are the foods I love. What fun is that? And although it's possible to follow the diet for a month or two or three, eventually I started craving the foods I've loved but that are now forbidden. This led to a sense that I was deprived, which only served to make the cravings stronger.

For most people that's the first thing that doom a diet even before it starts. Unless you've got more will power than eight draft horses, sooner or later you'll go back to the foods you love. Three months without a doughnut, eight months without a pizza, 14 months abstaining from fried chicken—it's got to get to you! And it almost always does.

There is another problem with deprivation that is even worse than what it does to your will power. Deprivation sets up two groups of food: "good" food (you know, stuff you're allowed, like turnips and bean curd) and "evil" food (you know, stuff you must never have like bacon and cashews). The result is that you begin to believe that many foods are actually your enemy, that your weight war is a battle between you and the evil food. This is very damaging—it places food in the wrong light. It twists your attitudes around and makes it much more difficult to come into any kind of balance with food or to place responsibility where it belongs.

With all of that in mind, I decided that whatever course of action I took, it would not deprive me of the foods I love.

2. Because of the deprivation, my diets caused resentment.

Being deprived of my favorite foods eventually caused me to resent my diet. After all those breakfasts of half a grapefruit and dry toast, after all those chocolate liquid lunches from cans, after all those skimpy dinners that taste as good as the cartons they came in, you start hating what you're eating. You long for the foods of the past. You go to lunch with friends, and while they're eating hamburgers you're grazing on a salad with low-fat dressing. ("Ah, those burgers sure look good. If only I weren't strapped to this diet I could be enjoying that food as well.")

Pretty soon, you start blaming the diet for everything:

> Why am I not enjoying my food? *The diet.*
> Why am I not having a good time? *The diet.*
> Why do I wish I were someone else? *The diet.*
> Why am I depressed? *The diet.*

You get the idea. The diet becomes the focal point for unhappiness. And that leads to resentment. **And any system that carries within it the seeds of resentment has a high likelihood of failure.**

So I decided that whatever I did would not carry the potential for resentment.

3. Diets are systems ripe with the possibilities of shame and guilt.

It's tough to be perfect. Despite my best intentions, there were times I found myself eating something I shouldn't have. I didn't actually *plan* to stop for ice cream—I just did. Or perhaps the only place open that evening was a fried chicken restaurant and, well, I had to eat something.

No matter what the excuse, I suspect that most dieters find themselves on the dark side of eating once in a while. The real problem comes afterwards: how do you handle the slip-up?

When I ate foods I shouldn't eat, I found myself feeling a bit ashamed, as if I were cheating on myself. That led to feelings of guilt and the sinking realization that I'd have to stick to my diet even more rigidly in the future, not to mention I'd have to spend an extra half-hour on the rowing machine just to work off that drumstick.

There's only one way to stop those feelings of shame and guilt during those diet side-trips: go off the diet! And that's exactly what happens to many dieters. They get tired of feeling ashamed or guilty, so they leave the diet behind.

In my view, any system that contains the seeds of shame and guilt is a system doomed to fail. Inevitably, those seeds will find fertile ground and bloom.

So I decided that whatever plan I came up with it wouldn't be one that held the potential for shame and guilt.

4. My diets were, by their very nature, temporary.

The crazy thing about many diets is that you set your goals, go on the diet, reach the goals and then go off the diet. But where does that leave you once you're done? You are, unfortunately, pretty much right back where you started. Your view of food hasn't changed nor has your attitudes about eating and your long-term behaviors. That means that, over time, you'll gain all that weight back.

I reasoned that what I needed was a new way of eating—a way I could live with the rest of my life, not just for a few months.

I knew that whatever the plan I came up with had to be permanent.

5. My diets didn't train me to eat less.

These days, we're facing a crisis in fat in this country these days. Over 55% of Americans are overweight. Obesity among children has reached on all-time high. Our food portions are totally out of control, and we eat food at every possible moment.

As I took a good, hard look at my eating habits, one thing was very clear: I was eating too much. Way too much. And I suspect that's why *most* individuals are too heavy. As a nation, we're eating far more than we need, and we've lost touch with eating in a reasonable way.

So if it's true that most overweight individuals are overweight because they eat too much, then it's obvious that we can't lose weight by changing *what* we eat. We have to change *how much* we eat. We have to reduce our portions and get in touch with the amount of food our bodies really need.

With this in mind, I decided that the new system I would used would show me how to reduce and manage my portions and bring me into a balance with food.

6. My diets didn't change my attitudes about food.

If anything, diets only worsened my attitudes about food. I saw food as either good or bad, and the more calories or fat something had, the worse it was. I began to resent that foods like Italian sausage and chocolate cake existed because I wanted them so much, and I equally resented that cauliflower and green beans existed because I felt condemned to eat them. The rules of my diets actually distracted me, making me think that the fault was with the food I was eating (or avoiding) and not with my own attitudes and habits.

My hunch was that to be successful over the long haul with weight loss, I had to develop new attitudes about eating and how I related to food. So with that in mind, I decided that whatever system I was going to use, it would promote new, positive attitudes about food.

7. Diets missed the point. **They called attention to the food, when the real problem was something within me, something much deeper and fundamental.**

Diets usually change the food one eats. But if the real problem with being overweight is *not* with food, then why to change the food one eats? No, if the real problem is with me, then *I've got to change ME!* That's the point my diets missed. They assumed that the problem was with the food. Wrong. Food is just food; it's not the problem. If I was going to have any success at all, I was going to have to work on changing me and my own approach to food.

8. Diets take away control.

Diets may be hard to do, but at least you don't have a lot of decisions to make. Diets come with calorie charts, fat charts, exchange tables, rules or regulations. If you want to know what to eat, just look on the charts. If you're not sure what to have for lunch, just look in column B. Simple, easy, and completely draining of power from you, because you're no longer in control. Somebody else is making the decisions for you, someone you probably don't even know. For me, the charts couldn't have known how much I liked cheeseburgers or Italian sausage. Nor could the charts understand why I was so unhappy.

From the time I was a little boy, I learned to give power away. The last thing I needed in my life was another place to relinquish more power. My new approach to eating had to include a way for me to be re-empowered, to gain back control of my eating.

That's Quite a Tall Order

So let's see—at this point, the new eating system I had to come up with required the following:

1. No deprivation.
2. No resentment.
3. No shame or guilt.

4. It has to be permanent.
5. It had to teach me to eat less food.
6. It had to change my attitudes about food.
7. It had to address the real problem: my relationship with food.
8. It had to give me back control of my eating.

Wow. All of that *and* no exercise as well. What kind of new system could I use that would meet all of these conditions?

The Answers

Attitudes

First things first: I had to develop a new set of attitudes about food. With my old attitudes, food was just a part of life, hardly worth a thought (except when no food was available!). I never considered how much food I really needed each day, what I thought about food or how I related to it. At 225 pounds, however, I sensed that I was out of balance with food and that I had to think long and hard about how food and I were going to coexist in the future.

The attitudes and principles covered in the chapter 6 are the ones I finally settled on. They have served me, my clients and my students very well in establishing a new outlook on food.

Portions

The next point I examined was: eating less. I knew I had to eat less food and that meant cutting back and controlling my portions. But that alone sounded pretty dismal. How could I be happy with a half a hamburger, a few French fries, just a little bit of coleslaw and no dessert? That doesn't sound like a meal! Won't I be hungry all the time and bitter about the little amount of food I'm eating?

Mindfulness

The solution to feeling satisfied with reduced portions came from a very ancient technique taught from the wisdom of the East. I had read about mindfulness some years ago and thought it would be helpful in my life but never put it into practice. Mindfulness is the moment-by-moment awareness of what we are doing. It's paying attention to what's going on and being aware of the activities of the present moment.

With mindfulness, I could eat my smaller portions carefully and attentively. My eating became slower, more thoughtful and appreciative. The smaller portions became more satisfying. And my new attitudes helped me feel better about food, to honor the food more and to honor myself more.

Control

When I put into practice the new attitudes, portions management and mindful eating, I had the freedom to look closely at how I was coming back into control of my eating. I could see that I had given away a lot of my power concerning food to other people and events and even food itself. Over time, I began to regain my control over what I ate, how much I ate, when I ate and what I enjoyed. The CAMP system was now an integrated part of my life.

These four main ingredients—Control, Attitudes, Mindfulness and Portions—gave the system its name: CAMP.

Together, these components create a powerful way for relating to food and eating.

The system allows you to eat the foods you want, so there are no feelings of deprivation.

With no deprivation in the system, no resentment occurs.

And with no resentment, there isn't any opportunity for shame and guilt.

The CAMP system is a way of eating that you can use for the rest of your life. It's permanent and you don't have to "go off the system" later on. Under the system, you'll learn to eat less. No matter what you eat, you'll take smaller amounts and enjoy them more that you ever did before. And when you eat less, you take in less energy and you give your body the opportunity to burn off stored energy reserves.

Finally, you'll discover that the CAMP system addresses the underlying causes of problems with food: control, power and relationships with food.

This book on the CAMP system will look at each of these elements in detail. The chapters ahead will give you step-by-step procedures for bringing the system into your life every day.

My Own Path

And as for my own experience with CAMP? I began the system in May, 1999, starting at a weight of 225 pounds. By the next January, eight months later, I had lost 60 pounds, amazingly down to 165. Nearly a year after that, I have managed and maintained that weight happily, looking forward to my new way of eating for the rest of my life.

The weight loss was wonderful. I never felt deprived or overly hungry, and the pounds came off slowly but steadily. It was almost as if my body was saying to me, "Finally! You got it right. I'll be more than happy to shed all these extra pounds I've been carrying around for years."

But as wonderful as the weight loss was, even better was the feeling that I had come into balance with food. I was eating for nourishment, for sustenance. After many years of giving control away, I was in control again. And I felt a real harmony with food—I knew that food and I were on the same side and we were working together for a healthy body, mind and spirit.

That's the real secret. When all of the elements of the CAMP system are working right, when you strike that harmony and balance, when you have married your commitment to your actions and your new attitudes to your intentions, then losing weight is no longer a goal. It is simply an extraordinary *byproduct* of the process. And *that* is the genuine miracle of the CAMP system.

3.

Basics of the CAMP System

There is nothing complicated, strange or mysterious about the CAMP system. It's not as if you have to eat pomegranates by the full moon or chew every bite of coleslaw 30 times while reciting the Declaration of Independence. No, the CAMP system uses simple, common sense ideas to achieve balance and harmony with food—ideas that all of us can use every day, for every meal, for every snack.

If there is any difficulty with the CAMP system, it is that most of us haven't learned how to slow down, wake up, pay attention and enjoy life. We're much too busy with our work, our kids, our relationships and our worries to be aware of life as it goes passing by.

The good news is that, through practice, we can all learn to slow down, wake up, pay attention and really enjoy life. We can, as the old saying goes, "take time to stop and smell the roses," a goal that most people would like to reach but don't know how to do so. The CAMP system will give you, step by step, a new path to follow, a way to "take time to stop and smell, taste and enjoy the food."

At the very center of the CAMP system is Control. This is the overall goal of the system, and it involves power over food.

All the other parts of the system are *pathways* to the goal of Control.

A Pathway Model of the CAMP System

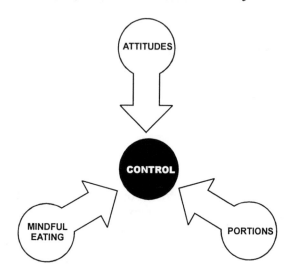

Attitudes. The first path to Control we'll consider in the CAMP system is Attitudes. Attitudes in the CAMP system include: respect for food, respect for self, and acknowledging the importance of living in dignity and grace, taking only as much food as is needed. The new attitudes of the CAMP system are covered in detail in Chapter 6.

Mindful Eating. Mindfulness is the state of being awake and alert, of paying attention to the world moment by moment. In the CAMP system, we give specific attention to food—its characteristics, origins, purposes and functions. As the second path to Control, Mindful Eating includes arrival, deliberateness, wakefulness, and awareness. An extensive discussion of mindfulness is in Chapters 7, 8, 9 and 10.

Portions. The third pathway to Control is Portions. Here you learn to manage how much you eat, bite by bite, chew by chew. This pathway includes boundaries, challenges, bite sizes and body awareness. Strategies, points of view and activities about portions are presented in Chapters 11, 12 and 13.

At each step of the way, you will gain more and more control over food, over your eating. Most of us have given away much of our power over food. In the CAMP system, you will grab that power back and take on your rightful, natural balance in dealing with food.

The core goal of the CAMP system, Control, is covered in Chapter 5 and includes:

- responsibility
- acceptance of consequences and outcomes
- non-blaming
- non-relinquishing
- power
- choices

In a Nutshell

As you read through the chapters ahead and do the practices there, the full CAMP procedure will be developed. Taking one skill at a time, you will gain mastery of the system and, by the time you get to chapter 14, you'll be ready for all the steps in the system.

In summary, though, here's what the CAMP system is all about.

You will learn:

- how to arrive at your meals.
- how to eat your food more thoughtfully, slowly, mindfully.
- how to determine the amount of food you really should be eating.
- how to seize back control of food.

As a result of these steps, you will come into harmony and balance with food.

During each meal, you will:

- eat slowly and carefully.
- be aware of your body and what it is telling you about the amount of food you're eating.
- know when to say 'enough' and stop eating.
- be attentive to the higher purpose of eating and live in more grace and dignity.

The CAMP system is not any more complicated than that.

4.

The CAMP Journal

The CAMP system is a discipline, an action plan, a new way of eating. Part of this system is to first get an idea of how much you're eating right now and then observe your eating habits change over the following weeks and months. One of the best ways to track your eating is to keep a diary or a Journal.

A Journal?!

No need to hide under the couch or grab a sharp weapon. This is not like a writing assignment in school. Basically, the CAMP Journal is going to be a record of what you're eating each day, a place to express your goals and your progress, and any other notes you want to add.

For Your Eyes Only

The best part is that no one else has to see your Journal—it's for your eyes only. That means that you don't have to write in complete sentences or worry about your best penmanship. This Journal is for you and you alone. It is your private account of your entire relationship with food. If you want to brag or cry or complain or whine, the Journal is ready to hear it all.

Your CAMP Journal doesn't have to be anything fancy. Buy yourself a spiral notebook or one of those black-and-white-marbled-cover composition books. Many bookstores also carry "blank books," which are very useful as journals. Find something that you like and make it your CAMP Journal. Decide right now that you can commit to writing in your Journal once each day for *at least the next 60 days.*

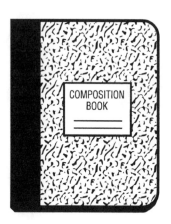

Reasons to Keep a CAMP Journal

I've heard comments from my students from time to time asking about the value of the Journal. Does it really matter that we write down everything that we eat every day?

Actually, it does! There are a number of benefits to keeping a CAMP Journal, and you should *not* take this lightly and decide to skip the Journal.

Here is why the CAMP Journal is important:

1. **It gives you a daily history of what you're eating, how much and where.** If you go on the CAMP system for a while and you're not losing weight, the answer to "why?" may be found by reviewing your Journal entries. Similarly, if things are working, you can use

your Journal as a record of what behaviors and strategies bring success.

2. **The Journal keeps you honest.** When you know that every bit of food you put in your mouth has to be recorded in your Journal, it may cause you to think twice about that extra snack or that second helping you didn't really need.

3. **The Journal adds another action to your eating plan.** It becomes a short ritual that helps reconfirm your commitment to the system.

4. **The Journal serves to remind you that your eating is an important activity.** Writing about eating is, in itself, a way of honoring your food. By keeping your Journal, you bring more sacredness to your eating.

5. **The Journal is one of many elements that foster mindfulness in your eating and about your eating.** Later on in this book you will learn about mindfulness, the moment-by-moment awareness of your life. By reserving a little time each day to write in your Journal, you pause and bring awareness to your eating. So the Journal is an important way of adding mindfulness to each day. If possible, make the process of writing in your Journal a time for quietness, reflection and calm. Devote your undivided attention to the Journal, if only for a few minutes. Begin to see the Journal as another opportunity to bring mindful moments into your life.

What Goes in the Journal?

The main function of your CAMP Journal is a daily record of what you've had to eat that day. You may decide to list the foods by meal, writing down what you had for breakfast, lunch, dinner, snacks, etc. Or you might prefer a single, long list of all the foods that day.

Along with listing the types of foods you had, you should also indicate something about how much of each food you ate. You don't have to measure out your food for this; instead, find a way of suggesting the size of each serving.

The sample entry from a Journal on the next page shows many examples of how to use terms suggesting food quantity without actually measuring food amounts. The sample page also gives you one idea of how you might set up your Journal.

Over the next weeks and months, your Journal will allow you to see shifts in not only the amount of food you're eating, but also the types of foods you're selecting. Also, your Journal will form a historical record of your changes as you develop a balance with food. The important thing here is to get in the daily habit of writing in your CAMP Journal, starting with the food you eat.

February 9, 2000

Breakfast
- *small glass of orange juice*
- *½ bagel with cream cheese*
- *¾ serving of cereal with 2% milk.*
- *cup of coffee*

Lunch
- *single cheeseburger*
- *large fries*
- *cola*

Dinner
- *two pieces of fried chicken*
- *large salad*
- *large serving of macaroni and cheese*
- *small piece of pie*
- *2 glasses of sweetened iced tea*

A sample Journal page. In this set-up, foods are listed by meals. You might also set yours up to record all the of the day's food in one long list.

Notice that for each entry there is some description of how much food was eaten.

Remember to include all foods and beverages in your Journal. Snacks are important. That candy bar you bought to eat on the ride home from work counts! The spoonful of mints you took as you left the restaurant last night should not be overlooked. It all adds up, and each bite or sip reflects the state of your relationship with food.

Other Entries

There are many other items you can put in your Journal as well. The journal can be a place to answer questions such as these:

- What am I discovering about food?

- What foods do I like? What foods am I *learning* to like or dislike?

- How are my food portions changing?

- What are my feelings about food? About myself? About my weight? About my control over food?

- What successes am I experiencing? How am I celebrating them?

- What failures do I experience? How I am dealing with those failures?

- What do I want to do better? How do I plan to make improvements?

If you enjoy writing, there's plenty to write about in your Journal. If you don't especially like writing, however, don't be overwhelmed by the list above. The Journal need not take much of your time and effort. The main thing is to "Keep it Simple." I put my Journal by my easy chair and spend only two or three minutes in the evening jotting down my foods of the day. Once in while I may have comments about events or discoveries that day, and I may take a little more time with the Journal. But usually I can complete the day's entry during a commercial break on a TV show.

Some of my students have found it easier to keep the Journal at the dinner table, completing entries as they happen. Experiment to find the best place to keep your Journal.

Two additional major items you can include in your Journal are:

- Goals and Milestones
- Weight

Goals and Milestones

Goals are important—they give you a good sense of where you want to be and when you want to get there. Goals serve as the road map of your program and tell you when you're on course or if you've gotten lost on a side trip. Just where would you like the CAMP system to take you? You might answer in terms of weight loss, a change in the size of your waistline or your coat size. You might just want to feel better about food and have more of a sense of well being after meals.

Goals can also be long-term or short-term. You might set goals for the week, for the month, for the year. The longer the goal, the more milestones you'll want to have to keep you on track.

Weight

The Journal is the ideal place to record your weight, and I encourage you to keep special track of it.

Some people don't like this idea and don't even own scales in their homes. I've heard some say, "I don't need a scale; I know from my belt size how I'm doing." Others just feel threatened by a scale, rather not knowing how much they weigh.

I've been there. I know what that feels like, and for many years I did not bother to get on the scales. But my own experience has taught me the value of tracking weight.

During my first months on the CAMP system, I was losing weight at the rate of 10 to 12 pounds a month. Oddly enough, however, I noticed almost no difference in how my clothes were fitting. If I had depended on my clothes to tell me how I was doing during that time, I would have been very discouraged and disappointed. In fact, I may have given up.

What kept me going was the fact that every week I saw two to four pounds disappear on my scales. This was very motivating.

I also learned that the number on my scales was not so much a value of my weight. It was actually a measure of how much I was in or out of harmony and balance with food. Don't think of your bathroom scales as a weight-measuring device—think of it as a balance-o-meter or a harmony-o-meter.

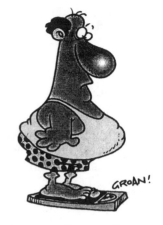

Putting the "Balance-O-Meter" to the Test

Decide on an "official weigh-in" day, perhaps once each week, and record your weight in your Journal. (Every Friday is my weigh-in day.) When your weight goes up or down or stays the same, take a good look at how much you're eating. See if you can identify any trends or explanations. Write the *whole* story of your recapturing harmony with food in your Journal, and use the Journal to keep track of your changing relationship with food and major or minor shifts in your thinking, preferences and tastes.

If You Miss a Day (or Two)

We all get very busy. There are a thousand distractions in every day, and it's difficult to remember to get it all done. Without doubt, there will be days when you climb into bed and suddenly think, "I didn't do my CAMP Journal today!"

Relax. There's no need to drag yourself up, grumble your way to the Journal and write about your food. Decide right now that it's okay to miss a day or so.

When you do miss writing in your Journal, just pick up when you can and continue. If there are gaps in your Journal, it doesn't matter. I've known students who thought that because they missed a day of writing that they couldn't continue with the Journal. Don't let a few missed days turn into an excuse to stop writing.

Red Flag

On the other hand, if you find yourself frequently forgetting to write, it's time to ask yourself about your commitment to the system. At a deep level, how important is weight reduction and management to you? How important is attaining harmony and balance with food? The Journal you haven't opened for a week is telling you something about yourself, your determination and what you consider to be significant.

It's Time

Even though I reached my target weight long ago, I continue to keep my Journal. Day by day, it beckons me, reminds me, keeps me attentive. It is a mirror of sorts, reflecting my changing tastes and habits and my new sense of balance. I have come to rely and depend on my Journal as a way of grounding myself and my eating behaviors. I invite you to commit to a Journal and realize the same benefits.

Don't skip this important step. Use your Journal as one of many indicators of your commitment to the program. Vow to keep it current each day.

Write your own story as you change your life and your relationship with food.

Practice - The Journal

At this point, stop. Go buy your Journal.

Begin recording each day what you're eating and some idea of how much.

Keep your Journal in a convenient place where you'll remember to do it each day. If you miss a day, don't worry about it. Just start writing again when you can.

Commit to keeping the Journal. You're in the process of changing all of your old habits, opinions, attitudes and values about food. Your Journal will be a contemporary and historical account of your journey. Don't skip it!

Eat normally for at least a week. Record the food each day without judgement. One week from now, come back to the book and continue with the next chapter.

Summary of Action steps

1. Buy the Journal.
2. Eat normally for at least a week.
3. Keep your Journal in a convenient spot.
4. Reserve quiet time each day to write in your Journal.
5. Record all meals in the Journal. Include what you ate as well as some idea of the amount of each food. Include meals, snacks, drinks, everything.
6. Record in your Journal any thoughts you have about food, the principles, yourself, what you like. Make this Journal a chronicle of your personal odyssey.
7. Record personal information in your Journal, such as your weight, belt size, dress size and waist size. Plan to update this information at least once each week.
8. State in your Journal your short-term goals and long-term goals. How much weight would you like to lose in a week? A month? By your next birthday? By next Fourth of July or Christmas? Set goals and milestones by writing them all down.
9. It's important that you gather information for about a week before going on. You'll get an idea of your current eating behavior and you'll get into the habit of writing every day. So when you have at least a week's worth of entries in your Journal, come back to the book and continue your adventure with the CAMP system.

Progress

At this point in the CAMP system you are:

☐ Keeping a daily Journal, recording your meals each day and any thoughts, ideas, insights and new points of view.

5.

Control

For 25 years, I handed my life over to a Little White Tube.

I couldn't go more than 40 minutes or so without grabbing the Little White Tube. I carried a Little White Tube with me wherever I went. The first thing in the morning was to find the Little White Tube. The last thing at night was to find the Little White Tube.

The Little White Tube robbed me of my health, my choices, my fun. And it did so with my full permission. I had relinquished my life to the Little White Tube. I was no longer in control.

In case you haven't guessed yet, the Little White Tube is a cigarette, and I was a willing addict to smoking for a quarter of a century. Only when I got ready to quit did it occur to me how much power I had turned over to tobacco. And only when I was really ready to grab back that power could I quit smoking and stay quit.

Later, when it came to my own issues about eating, it didn't surprise me to consider that during most of my life I had probably given up similar control over food. It meant that I had to be ready to grab back my power of food. Only then could I successfully change my eating behaviors.

Power and Choices

During the course on the CAMP system, I ask my students to write and finish this sentence in their journals. If you'd like to see how your answer compares with theirs, you can do the exercise as well. Here is the sentence:

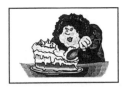

"When I overeat,

I overeat because _____."

Go ahead and take a moment to think how you would finish that sentence. Then, read on to discover how others have finished it and what their answers reveal.

Control in our lives takes two distinct forms: Power and Choices.

Power refers to what we allow to influence us. When we are overweight or underweight, we have chosen to give power over food away to someone or something else. This is convenient and absolves us of responsibility.

Choices are those conscious and unconscious decisions made about food. When we are overweight or underweight, we let others make choices for us, or we allow our unconscious minds to make decisions. This takes much less work than making our own deliberate and mindful decisions.

When you <u>do not</u> have control over food:

- You give away power by assigning blame to other things for your overeating.
- You let others make decisions for you about food.
- You allow your auto pilot to make important determinations about when you eat and how much you eat.

When you <u>have</u> control over food:

- you grab back and keep the power you've given away
- you stop allowing others to make choices for you

- you stop making *mindless* choices and begin making *mindful* choices.

Power Issues

Here are some answers people commonly give to the question, "When I overeat, I overeat because _____."

"When I overeat, I overeat because ..."	Comments
...of my family & relationships."	We blame our spouses, parents, kids, lovers, cousins, whoever is convenient. One of my clients said she overate because when she visited her mother her mother insisted that she eat lots of food every meal. And, well, she couldn't say no to her mom.
...of my job."	Most of us experience high stress on the job. We have little control of how and when we work, we may have tyrants for bosses, and the deadlines keep on coming. Food is one way of getting through the day. And then, there's always food in the office—snacks, office parties, business lunches and celebrations all have lots of food and plenty of temptation. And, well, you just *have* to eat what people bring in!
...of events in my life."	Every celebration has food with it: birthdays, holidays, parties, even illnesses and deaths. And, well, you don't want to be a party pooper and not eat!
...I seek pleasure."	Sometimes you just want to feel good and to taste something good. Besides, don't you deserve it for putting up with everything else life throws at you?

"When I overeat, I overeat because ..."	Comments
...I can't resist the food."	It doesn't matter how rich or mighty you are. Everyone, from the most powerful to the very weakest in our society, can be overpowered by a candy bar or a bag of potato chips. So what chance do you have? Might as well give into the lure of food.
...I have health problems or imbalances."	Some recent diets on the market have proposed that individuals can be addicted to carbohydrates. I'm not stating any opinions about this claim, but I've seen students conveniently blame their overeating on their perceived addiction. Their logic is: "I have an addiction. Therefore, I'm completely out of control and must overeat." I've also had clients who have said, "I can't lose weight—my metabolism is too slow." Again, very convenient, don't you think?
...I want to reward myself for something."	We learn early in our lives that food is a reward (and, perhaps, that food was withheld as punishment). I remember the good old days when I was dieting and doing exercises. I'd eat well all week and get my exercises in three or four times in a week. So how did I celebrate this behavior? By going out on the weekend and eating a big meal at a restaurant. I saw it as my reward for being a good boy. I might as well not have even bothered with the diet.
...I want to feel better about something."	We look to food to correct and smooth over the states of boredom, sadness, loneliness, feeling of failure and low self-esteem. We expect food to fill the vacancies in our emotional lives. After all, won't chocolate mend the hurt of an angry boyfriend or girlfriend? Won't a doughnut boost the self image? And is there anything better for melancholy than a bag of potato chips?

"When I overeat, I overeat because ..."	Comments
...I was trained to eat the wrong foods."	This is one of my favorites. For a long time, I believed my eating problem was that I learned as a child to enjoy the wrong types of foods. So it wasn't my fault that I liked fried chicken and sausage. These are tastes that developed in my childhood and are the legacy of the early lessons of my history. Don't blame me.
...I don't have the time to devote to a better relationship with food.	Far and away this excuse is the most popular. "I want to do better, but I don't have the time." We blame the clock, reasoning if there could only be a few extra hours in the day, *then* we'd have time to devote to better eating.

Did you find your own answer somewhere in those statements?

Actually, you probably recognized *several* familiar statements there. Depending on where you may be in your life, you will use a variety of rationalizations to justify your eating behaviors.

The Uncomfortable but Unavoidable Powerful Truth

The truth is that there is only one 'correct' way to finish the statement "When I overeat, I overeat because_____." There is only one answer that accurately pins the blame where it belongs, only one answer that precisely focuses attention on the real cause. Ready? Okay, here it is:

"When I overeat, I overeat *because I choose to.*"

That's it. Never mind all the reasons and excuses. Never mind that you're lonely or happy or at a party or your mother fed you too much as a child. Overeating is a choice we make. No one else can be blamed; the responsibility cannot be passed on.

If you go back and reread the excuse statements in this chapter, think of each of them as giving away power.

When you say...	*...it means...*
"I overeat because of my family"	You are giving power away to other people.
"I overeat because of my job."	You are giving power away to your livelihood, your coworkers, your boss.
"I overeat because I want to reward myself."	You are giving power away to your low self-esteem.
"I overeat because I want to feel better about something.	You are giving power away to food as a provider of comfort.
"I overeat because I wasn't taught to eat correctly."	You are giving power away to your history.
"I overeat because I just can't resist the food."	Power is being given away to food as an object of addiction.
"I overeat because I don't have time to do better."	Power is being given away to the clock.

Get the idea? Every excuse you give is another way you give up your power to some outside agent.

Another Truth

An important truth of the CAMP system is that our overeating is a sign that we have a major imbalance in our lives. This imbalance is not only physical; indeed, overeating is an indication that we are out of balance in mind and in spirit as well.

When we overeat, we eat without thinking—we eat *mindlessly*. We take food for granted and fail to consider its gifts. We can eat an entire meal and have absolutely no memory of it as soon as we're done. Worse, we don't even know how much we've eaten.

When we overeat, we switch our spirits off. We stop appreciating food and the miracle of eating. We allow our spirits to be distracted out of the present moment and we fail to arrive at a balance and harmony with food. We turn our backs on living more in a sacred way, with more grace and dignity.

Is it any wonder that most diets fail?

- Any program to correct problems with eating that ignores the mental and spiritual parts of the problem has little chance of success.
- Any program that focuses on the number of calories in food but ignores the mind and spirit of the person who struggles cannot have lasting achievement.

When one comes into balance with food, the relationships of food to body, mind and spirit are equal.

Food feeds the body, gives it sustenance, provides energy and helps the body repair itself

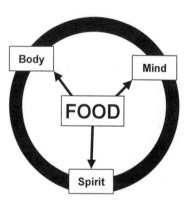

Food feeds the mind, stimulates the senses, provides opportunity for thought and reflection.

Food feeds the spirit, raises consciousness, uplifts appreciation, brings mindfulness.

When all are in *balance*, they act in *harmony*. Their connection (shown as a black ring) is a perfect circle.

No More Excuses

How do you give up your power? What excuses do you use? When you find yourself overeating, what's going through your mind to justify it to yourself? In what ways do these thoughts spin you out of control with food?

As overeaters, somehow along the way we have lost—no, freely relinquished—our power over food. It's all too easy. "Don't blame me if I overeat! It's the fault of my boss / mother / addiction / kids / loneliness / boredom / anger." We think the payoff is that food will somehow fix everything that is wrong. We forget that there is a terrible price to pay—a penalty that shows up on the bathroom scales and on our ever-shrinking belts.

To accept the full responsibility for overeating is to begin to grab back all the power you've given away. And the first step towards this goal is to stop making excuses. The bad news I bring you is that you can no longer blame anyone or anything else for your overeating. From this moment on, those excuses are history; they just don't cut it any more. Want to blame your family or your spouse for your overeating? Sorry. Are you convinced that your job drives you to eat more? Won't work. Remember: the reason that you overeat *is that you choose to*. Period.

The good news is that when you stop making excuses, you immediately receive a huge chunk of power you haven't had. Just as you choose to overeat, you can choose to come into balance with food.

The Parable of Sue

Sue was aware that she didn't have much control over her eating, but there were good reasons. She had a long commute to work, and recently her office moved so she had plenty of extra work to do. Her husband recently went into the hospital for heart surgery, so she was busy with him, getting to the hospital and making sure the kids were being cared for. As much as she wanted to, she couldn't find the time to concentrate on eating well.

Then one day, Sue was at the grocery store shopping for several weeks' worth of food. It was a Saturday morning, and the store was full of shoppers. Somewhere in the middle of the sugar and flour aisle, Sue noticed that the stone in her wedding ring was missing. It had fallen out of the setting. Sue stopped in her tracks; her mind raced. "Was the stone in the ring when I came into the store?" she asked herself. The diamond was large and valuable, and had sentimental value as well—it came from the wedding ring of her husband's grandmother.

Without any more thought, Sue abandoned her food cart and began looking for the ring. She looked over every inch of floor she had walked. She searched through all the fruits and vegetables she might have handled. No shelf, box, can or item escaped her eye. Her schedule for the rest of the day no longer mattered. The noise and busyness of the store did not distract her from her goal. That stone, that lost valuable, priceless diamond was the only important thing.

Now, what's the point here? Just what is the difference between Sue's approach to food and eating and her approach to the missing ring. Sue decided that the missing stone was valuable, and once she decided that, nothing could get in her way of finding it. Notice that she didn't say, "Well, I could look for the diamond, but it's so busy in here and I'm running late and I have too much to think about ..."

And yet, those are exactly the excuses Sue makes about not finding ways to improve her relationship with food. Obviously, Sue made the *decision* that food issues just weren't that important. Once she decided that, she could allow all sorts of excuses to explain why she didn't give more time or effort to her eating.

Where are you in your life? Is your relationship with food *important* to you yet? Is it a precious gem in your ring? Are you ready to search for balance and harmony with food in the same way you'd search for a missing diamond?

The lesson that Sue teaches us is that making something important or valuable is a *choice*. You can, right now, as you read this, make a decision to view your relationship with food as a top priority in your life.

Choices

The other aspect of control is making conscious decisions. Every act of eating is a choice you make. These choices include:

- the type of food you eat
- where you eat
- when you eat
- how often you eat
- the amount of food you eat
- the size of the bite you chew
- how fast or slowly you chew

- how thoroughly you chew your food
- when you swallow it
- how much time you take between bites
- when you stop eating

and on and on. For most of these choices, we're not even aware we are making them. They are automatic and habitual and *mindless*. Years of unconscious decisions add up to the point where we gain weight and wonder why. After all, we think, we didn't *choose* to gain weight, did we?

A Simple Food Economy

The Simple Food Economy shown here speaks to the idea of choices.

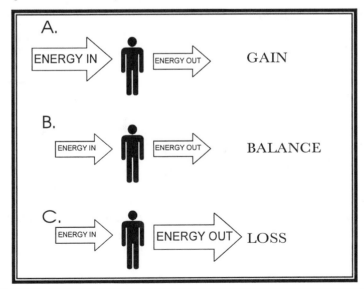

In diagram A, more food energy is coming in than is being used. Weight gain is the result.

In diagram B, there is a balance of energy in and out. Weight will not change.

In diagram C, there is more energy being used up than food energy coming in. Weight loss is the result.

At first this diagram looks too simple. After all, isn't it obvious that if you eat more than you need, you'll gain weight? As I got deeper and deeper into the CAMP way, though, I realized that this diagram is all about choices. With every bite, you make choice—a decision (whether you're aware of it or not)—about how you want to relate to food and its energy.

If you take in more energy than you use, you gain weight (diagram A at the top). This is where most overeaters find themselves. They eat for pleasure, for punishment, for social reasons, or for dozens of other excuses. They choose to ignore the messages of their bodies, *eating far more than their bodies need.* I spent many years at diagram A. Only after coming to the CAMP system did I realize that I was *choosing* to dwell in diagram A, seriously out of balance with food and eating. I knew then that I could *choose* to be in any part of this economy I wanted.

If you take in less energy than your use, you lose weight (diagram C at the bottom). **Like it or not, if you want to lose weight you have to spend some time here.** One way is to increase your body's furnace by exercising, which elevates your metabolism and the rate at which you burn food. Or you can reduce your portions, cutting back on the amount of energy you bring into your system. When the body cannot find energy in the digestive tract, it looks for energy elsewhere. Actually, your body is pretty smart—it knows exactly where it has stored food and how long that fat has been there. By eating less than you burn, you force your body to seek out and use stored fat. If you want to lose weight, this is where you want to be, and trick is to eat *just a little* less than you need. Weight loss is slow but sensible as you come more and more into harmony with food.

When I started eating the CAMP way, I realized that I had to stay in diagram C each day. If I felt a little hungry during the day, I took it as a sign that my body was shifting its focus from the food I ate to the food I stored (fat). So a little hunger was a good sign; I enjoyed it. When the hunger got strong or my thoughts turned to food often, I knew it was time to eat. But—and here's the real core of this message—*I felt I was in control*. At last, truly in control. By placing myself in diagram C and choosing to stay there, I was telling my body: "Go ahead. Burn off that excess fat. This is the way I'm going to get back into balance." The pounds came off, sometimes three or four each week. My body was answering back: "Aha! You finally got it. Let me get rid of all this extra weight and let's get back to some common sense with food."

If you take in as much energy as you use, you maintain weight (diagram B in the middle). Once you feel you're at the weight your body wants to be (whatever that means to you), your job is to find what your balance is between energy in and energy out. Only you know what that means. No chart or book or doctor or diet guru knows what your life is like, what your needs are or what your balance is.

When I reached the weight I thought I should be, I had to experiment quite a bit to find the balance. I ate more each day and still lost a little weight. Slowly, I increased the amount I ate until my weight stabilized.

It may take you months or even years to get to that point. No matter. The victory isn't months or years away; rather, it's day by day, meal by meal. If today you're overweight *but* you're in balance with food, then the battle has been won!

Any time of the day or night, you can place yourself somewhere on this food economy. When you sit down to eat, you can decide where you want to be. With each bite you take, you make a choice. This is power of knowing about this food economy. If you overeat, it's your choice. If you eat less and allow your body to burn up stored food, it's your choice. When you decide you stay in balance with food, it's your option.

With every bite we take, we make a decision of where we want to be in this economy. Granted, most of our decisions are unconscious, but they are <u>our</u> decisions nonetheless.

We will return to the Simple Food Economy later on when we tackle the topic of portion sizes. For now, the idea is to begin to see yourself somewhere in this economy. In which part of the diagram (A, B or C) do you normally dwell? Realize that you are wherever you are because of the *choices* you make.

Recapturing Power

The CAMP system is about recapturing control over food, and the system will give you tools, strategies and approaches for doing just that. The first place to start is to identify and become aware of

- the excuses you make
- the ways you give up power
- the opportunities that come your way to grab control back.

Your Journal will be the first line in plotting your own course of finding yourself and the power you've given away.

Practice - Control

In this chapter, you took an in-depth look at the "C" of CAMP—Control. You saw the common ways that people give up power, lose control over food, and stop making conscious choices.

You can begin to make progress in recovering your own control over food by using your Journal. At this point, you should be recording the food you're eating every day. You should also be using your Journal to jot down your thoughts about food and your relationship to it.

Starting now, add more to your Journal. During the time you're writing in your Journal, take a good look at your day and at your eating behaviors.

Ask yourself:

- Did I overeat at all?
- What excuses do I make for overeating?
- When I make excuses, who is really getting my power?
- Why do I give up my power? How does it benefit me?
- In what ways could I begin to grab control back?

- Look over what you ate each day and then ask yourself: "Where did I dwell today in my food economy? In diagram A, B or C?"

As answers come to you, add them to your Journal. They won't all come at once. This is a slow process. But keep at it.

Review the Simple Food Economy diagram. Sketch it in your Journal (it doesn't have to be any work of art!). What does that diagram teach you or what do you think about when you see it? Day by day, where are you in that diagram? At A? B? C? Jot down your thoughts in your Journal.

Finally, review the diagram showing the balance of body, mind and spirit relative to food. Write your thoughts on this as well. How much in or out of balance are you? Are you using food for sensation? to lift your moods? to punish yourself? What are you overlooking? List some simple ways you could achieve better balance.

Give yourself at least several days of normal eating and Journal writing before going on to the next chapter. And remember: if you don't like writing in the Journal, write what you can. The most important thing is to write something every day. But as much as possible, don't skip this step. Coming to grips with control issues is vital to success in the CAMP system.

Becoming aware of our control issues is an important first step in regaining control. But it is only a step. The rest of this book sets a course to help you do serious work in recapturing your control.

There are *three main paths* to recovering personal power and control over food:

- Attitudes (chapter 6)
- Mindful Eating (chapters 7 through 10)
- Portions (chapter 11 through 13)

As your **attitudes** change, your control comes more and more into alignment.

As you learn to eat **mindfully**, you can gain power over food bite by bite.

As you acquire strategies about **portions**, your sense of balance, harmony and control over food can return, strong and potent.

Ahead, you'll be eating for *you*—not anyone or anything else. You'll be allowing food to nourish you, replenish your mind, refresh your spirit. This is the essence of CAMP.

Progress

At this point in the CAMP system you are:

❑ Continuing your daily food Journal.

❑ Becoming aware of where you've given up control of food and recording what you've learned in your Food Journal.

❑ Placing yourself on the Food Economy diagram each day, each meal, even each bite.

6.

Attitudes

 Over the last five years or so I've worked with hundreds of people in Quit Smoking programs. I give them dozens and dozens of strategies for quitting. I tell them how to fight cravings and identify their triggers. With great care I inform them about what will undermine their efforts and what steps to take to avoid that sabotage.

But the best advice I give them is that they have to *change their attitudes* about smoking. Like anything in life, attitudes are 90% of the game. Those who can change their attitudes about smoking have the greatest chance of success in quitting.

Coming to grips with food is no different. Attitudes matter. The new attitudes of the CAMP system are based on ten broad principles (shown on the next page). These large ideas set the stage for a new and powerful mental approach to eating, food and relationships to food. Attitudes are the first path to personal control and power over food.

The CAMP System

Ten Principles

1. Never feel deprived.

2. Food is for nourishment—sustenance for body, mind and spirit.

3. All food is special and merits our deepest respect— it is a great gift of energy and effort.

4. There will always be more food.

5. In a land of abundance, there is never a reason to be overweight.

6. It is far better to leave some food uneaten than to eat more than is needed.

7. Hunger can be an ally, a sign that the body is adjusting and coming back into balance.

8. "Success" with food has more to do with harmony with food rather than weight loss.

9. If we learn to tune in to the body and trust it, it will tell us when we are in balance and harmony with food.

10. Being in harmony and balance with food is part of living a life of dignity and grace.

When we were very little children, it was extremely easy for us to believe new ideas, new fantasies, new "let's pretend." With the power of our imagination and the willingness to believe, we could turn ordinary objects into magical items. If we wanted to, we could believe that a simple stick was a shining sword ready for battle. With just a little effort, an old cardboard box could magically become a kitchen stove ready to prepare tea for a tea party.

As adults, we often forget those magical days of our youth. But the magic is still there—if we want to, we can accept new ideas simply by choosing to believe them.

And this is what I would like you to do with these ten new principles of the CAMP system. In many cases, accepting the ideas in these principles may be just as easy as deciding to believe in them. In other cases, it may take you a lot of time and thought to eventually adopt the ideas here. For that reason, *it's important to review the ten principles at least once every day.*

For now, let's take a close look at each of these principles and what they can mean to us in our new way of looking at food.

1. Never Feel Deprived

The first and foremost principle of the CAMP system is to never feel deprived. This means that all foods are available to you. There is no need to crave any particular food because all foods are available to you. Now, this doesn't mean that you eat nothing but cake morning, noon and night. We want to use common sense. But it does mean that if you feel you must have a certain food, you should go ahead and have some of the food.

Here is what I've found: when you decide to never be deprived, you feel free to consider all foods. Since nothing is forbidden, no foods become the object of intense craving. And often just a small amount of food is enough to satisfy the urge to eat it.

2. Food is for nourishment—sustenance for body, mind and spirit.

These days, food is so abundant, so plentiful and in such variety that we have forgotten what it's really all about. Have you ever noticed that almost any kind of celebration involves food? Why is it that we can't go to a movie theatre and just enjoy the movie without food? You can buy almost any type of food now in snack size, meal size, jumbo size and Godzilla size. We are constantly bombarded with advertisements about food that try to convince us that we should be eating great quantities all the time in any place for any reason.

And we are so clever in thinking up reasons to eat. We eat to celebrate, to commemorate, to welcome, to say goodbye, to mourn, to chase the blues, to meet with friends, to help get the sale, to plan, to hide, to punish ourselves, to watch a ballgame, to have a reunion, to be polite, and on and on and on. Lost in all of this is the true value of food—as nourishment and to replenish our energy.

The time has come to return to those values and put food in the proper perspective. If you are heavier than you want to be, you've been eating for many of the reasons mentioned above. The new attitude in the CAMP system is that *food is for nourishment*—nourishment for body and purpose. Food should enhance our lives, not weaken them. If you leave a meal feeling stuffed, bloated, and uncomfortable, you've not only eaten too much—you've also allowed food to undermine your sense of well being and purpose and you've probably eaten that extra food for the wrong reason.

Here is what I've found: when you see food primarily for nourishment, you begin to get in the habit of asking yourself, "Do I really need this food?" When the answer to that question is "no," it becomes more and more likely that you won't eat food you don't really need. Instead, you will increase your control over food and your eating.

3. All food is special and merits our deepest respect—it is a great gift of energy and effort.

If we had lived thousands of years ago, we would know all the efforts it took to bring food to our mouths. We would know who killed the food, who carried it, who prepared it, who grew it and who tended to it. Food was scarce, and a meal was a great and special event. Having cornmeal wasn't just "Oh, just another helping of cornmeal." You would have had a sense of how hard it was to get that corn, how you felt when the rains almost didn't come, how you had to wait for the corn to be ready on the ears, how you had to grind the corn, make the fire, bake the food. You may have remembered a frightening, hungry time when there wasn't enough cornmeal to go around. So mostly you felt humble and grateful that food was available.

But today, we're so far removed from the origin of our food that we no longer appreciate how special it is. Our supermarkets are full of food in unimaginable varieties. Restaurants and fast food outlets pepper our roadways. Convenience stores now beckon us with every gas fill-up. To put meat on the table is a simple act we take for granted; rarely do we consider how long it took to raise the animal, what food was necessary, how the animal was slaughtered, transported and prepared. Whole generations have now grown up thinking that hamburger is just brown stuff that comes from the market. When I taught high school biology my students were appalled to learn that hamburger is actually cow muscle! "Eeeeeuuuu," they would say.

Clearly, our society takes food for granted. And when we do that, it's easy to eat at every opportunity.

The third principle of the CAMP system is to see food as something extremely special. Food isn't to be taken lightly—rather, it is the substance that gives us life. When we learn to see food as special, as exceptional, even as sacred, it becomes much more difficult to scarf down those big meals and gulp down all those snacks and sweets as if they were water. Instead, each encounter with food becomes a distinctive event, one that we take seriously and respectfully.

Here is what I've found: when I treat food with the utmost respect, I can't eat it carelessly. That would be like dancing on an altar. If you believe an altar is a sacred place, you'd never think of dancing there. And if you think food is very special, you reach a point where you don't want to misuse or abuse it.

If I gave you a bottle of nitroglycerine and told you to rush it up three flights of stairs, you might be nervous. After all, nitroglycerine is a very unstable, explosive substance. The slightest misstep might end in disaster. You would carry the bottle carefully, mindful of your every step, your every movement. You would slow down, take your time and be aware of what you're doing. Nitroglycerine in the bottle is very dangerous, and you would show it the respect it deserves. (Oddly enough, the same nitroglycerine, used in small quantities as medicine, has healing properties and helps the heart.)

We need to see food in the same way. Food, handled with care in reasonable quantities, is the source of life. But mishandled, food can be very dangerous. When we don't see food as special, as deserving of our honor, we tend to misuse it. And, like nitroglycerine, food mishandled can have a devastating effect on us.

Seeing food as special, important, even sacred, isn't difficult. All you have to do is *decide* to see food that way. Over time, your attitudes about food will shift to view food that way all the time.

This new view of food applies to *all* foods. The CAMP system sees all types of foods as equally valuable, as great gifts of energy and effort. This new attitude forces us out of the mindset that green beans are "good" and brownies are "bad." Beans are beans and brownies are brownies, both with wonderful gifts of sustenance and flavor. It's how we eat those foods—mindlessly or mindfully, with honor or with disregard—that makes the big difference in how food enters our lives and affects us.

4. There will always be more food.

This seemingly simple sentence has profound implications for how we eat. It means that you don't have to eat huge meals, that you don't have to finish your plate, that you don't have to stuff yourself to the point of immobility. It means that you might put a small amount of food on your plate to begin with. If, when you finish that food, you still want more, you can *always go get more*. Astonishing. It means that in a restaurant, you might order of small amount of food to begin with and later, if you want more food, you can *always order more food*. Amazing!

Somewhere, deep within the ancient reptilian part of our brain, we have what I call the "gorge reflex." This is the part of the brain that gets very excited when it senses the presence of a lot of food. At a buffet, for example, the gorge reflex can kick in and convince us that we have to eat all the food we see in front of us. All of it. (The next time you're at a buffet, notice how people are loading up their plates, as if they are compelled to eat every scrap of food they see. They must be in the irresistible grip of the reptilian gorge reflex!) The fourth principal of the CAMP system tells us that we can enjoy food today, and that there will always be food another day—we don't have to eat it all now.

Here is what I've found: when I know that I can always have food at a later time, I find myself eating less. I can pass by that ice cream in the freezer, knowing it will be there tomorrow, and that I can have some tomorrow. I know in a restaurant that I don't have to order the pizza or the steak every time; the next time I'm in that restaurant those foods will be there and available. The core idea of this fourth principal is extremely liberating—it gives me freedom and control, as I know the foods I love will always be there for me when I want and when I decide to have them.

5. In a land of abundance, there is never a reason to be overweight.

Principle #5 seems to be the opposite of what one would expect. After all, wouldn't it make more sense to say that in a land of abundance there are many reasons to be overweight? Let's take a closer look.

If we lived in a land where food was scarce, those who would survive the best would be those who could eat a lot of food during the rare times that food was available. The idea would be to fatten up during the times that food was plentiful so you could survive the times when food was difficult to get, living off of your own reserves.

On the other hand, we live in a land where food is amazingly abundant. For most of us, getting food any time of the year is no problem. There are no scarce times. The most we have to eat at any meal should be just enough to get us to the next meal. And this is a very important way that we honor the food we have—to eat just what we need to get us to the next meal and to the next day.

Here is what I've found: remembering that food is forever abundant has made it easier for me not to overeat. There is no reason for me to fatten up. With so much food around, I could concentrate on seeing food as nourishment and not as something to stockpile. At home, I can take a small serving of food knowing that there will be more if or when I need it. At a restaurant, I can order a small amount fully aware that if I need more I can always order more. At the buffet, I know that I don't have to taste everything—the buffet will be there the next time when I can enjoy some of the other foods there.

6. It is far better to leave some food uneaten than to eat more than is needed.

Of all the principles in the CAMP system, this is the one with which people have the most problems. It's actually unthinkable for some people to leave food on their plates. When I was young, my father reminded me to think of the "starving Armenians" before I considered leaving food on my plate. (I never could figure out exactly how eating all my food would help those starving Armenians, but usually I ate all my food anyway.)

We learned in Principle #3 that all food is a great gift of energy and effort. If that is true, then we must honor the food have. When we accept that gift for nourishment of body, mind, and spirit, we give food the honor it deserves. When we eat more than we need, however, we dishonor the gift—we take it for granted, and we devalue the energy and effort to produce it.

So, sometimes you have to throw away the food you don't eat. This is difficult, because it seems so wasteful. And indeed it may be a little wasteful. But it's far better to waste some of the food rather than eat food we don't need. It's odd how we detest putting perfectly good food in the trash can, but we think it's fine to put that food in our bodies instead, even when we don't need the food. If it helps, think of throwing food away as a means of giving some of the gift back to the universe. You are returning the food you don't need back to the earth that created it.

Here is what I've found: when we eat more than we actually need, we cross a boundary of the spirit, of the heart. We lose our sense of appreciation for the food. When we eat for reasons other than for nutrition, we abandon the acknowledgement of the gift of food and, by so doing, we trivialize the gift.

7. Hunger can be an ally, a sign that the body is adjusting and coming back into balance.

Diets fail for many reasons, and one of them is that people are afraid to feel hunger. When I dieted, I always resented feeling hungry. It was a constant reminder that I wasn't getting the foods I loved, and that, well, I might just starve to death if I can't get more food!

Needless to say, I didn't starve, but you can be sure the diet didn't last long.

And yet, if you're going to lose weight, you have to reach a point where your body is going to start burning the stored food you've been carrying around. And that will usually involve some feelings of hunger.

Another important new attitude of the CAMP system is that *some* hunger is okay. Right now, when you feel hunger signals, you're probably used to thinking, "I've got to get something to eat!" The CAMP system, however, sees hunger differently.

When you're hungry, your body is going to look for food in your digestive system. If it doesn't find much there, it will start to burn off stored food. *And this is what you want.*

Here is what I've found: First, I learned that what I usually called "hunger" was just a little *emptiness*. That so few of us have every *really* been hungry to the point of malnutrition or starvation is a blessing, and we have to guard against confusing an empty stomach with genuine hunger.

I also learned to consider hunger (emptiness) a friend. I came to know that hunger was my body burning stored food and to just enjoy it. If ever I felt really strong hunger, I didn't pause even for a second in getting a snack. But most of the time, if I just let hunger take its course I was fine—I never found myself weak on the floor ready to pass out from lack of food. Amazing, isn't it?

When you're a little hungry, it means that <u>the system is working</u>. You can't lose weight if you don't force your body to burn excess fat.

8. "Success" with food has more to do with harmony with food rather than weight loss.

What does success with food mean to you? Your first answer might be "losing weight," but you might want to think deeper.

I believe that most people with weight problems are that way because, at some fundamental level, they have gotten out of balance with food. Diets don't do much good in such cases, because changing the food we eat doesn't necessarily bring us back into balance. No, to fix what is wrong we have to go down to that fundamental level and find that balance with food again.

Success with the CAMP system, therefore, means getting in touch with the role food plays in our lives, getting back into balance with food and then living in a harmonious relationship it.

What I have found out: when people get into balance with food, weight loss and weight management occur as amazing byproducts of the process. The real trick is to set our goals towards *balance* rather than towards weight loss

9. If we learn to tune in to the body and trust it, it will tell us when we are in balance and harmony with food.

Our bodies are very smart. They know the foods that are best for us, and they know how much food is appropriate. We have learned, however, to ignore the messages our bodies give us, instead relying on other people, other voices and, in a big way, advertisers to tell us what's right for us.

It's time to change that and start listening to our own bodies again. It's as if we've all been listening to the wrong radio station all these years. We have to tune in our own radio stations, turn the antenna and listen to— and trust—the internal voice.

The techniques in the CAMP system will give you the time and the opportunity to slow down and listen to your own body. Slowly, you can learn to identify the foods right for you and what quantity of food makes sense for you.

This is the essence of living in harmony and balance with food. Here, *harmony* means that we have a sense of eating the right things in the right proportions for ourselves. It is an attitude that we are in cooperation with food, that we show food the respect it deserves and it, in turn, treats us well.

The term *balance* indicates a sense that our food needs match our food portions and that food is equally feeding body, mind and spirit. We fully accept food as nourishment. We eat what we need, not more and not less.

What I have found out: An essential part of mindfulness is paying close attention to our bodies and what they tell us. We have to make the effort to stop and listen carefully. If we can do that, the lessons we learn are profound.

10. Being in harmony and balance with food is part of living a life of dignity and grace.

When I realized that I had to lose weight, I got a picture in my mind. It was a powerful picture of myself, and it stayed with me during the many months I was losing weight. This picture helped me to stay on track, reminding me constantly of where I was and where I wanted to be.

The picture I saw was of my old self and what I must have looked like while I was eating. I saw myself stuffing food into my face without any thought or appreciation. I saw a slob who somehow lost sight of what it meant to live with a sense of grace. I imagined myself with food all over my mouth and down my chin, with food crumbs on my chest and all over my lap. Whether or not this picture was accurate is not important. The power of the picture, however, was that I didn't like what I saw.

I had another picture in mind at the same time. I imagined what a person would look like who lived with dignity about food. In this picture, the person would eat only what he needed. He would eat the food slowly and with care. When he was full and had what he needed, he would stop eating. He was gentle and kind with himself. He treated food with respect and the food repaid him with equal kindness.

This, too, was a powerful picture, and it was one I liked. I wanted to be that person, and I came to realize that *I could become that person*. I knew that when I got into harmony and balance with food, I could live my life with more grace and dignity, and that this goal was one of the highest aims to which humans could aspire.

What I have found out: If we set out to lose weight, we've got it wrong. If we set out to come into balance, to live in harmony, to increase the dignity in our lives, then weight loss and management arises naturally and spontaneously, flowing out of our higher selves and becoming a permanent part of who we are.

Conclusion

These Ten Principles are for you. They will speak to each person differently, but as you read them and re-read them, you will find how they speak to your own truth.

Also, as you read them again and again, they will become part of your belief system. You will accept them as valid ideas and find ways to bring them to your own eating.

This, in turn, will give you more power and control over your eating. *You* will decide when you leave food on your plate. *You* will decide how to deal with slight feelings of hunger. *You* will define success for yourself. You will tune in to your body and learn to trust it.

These are all control issues, and by accepting the principles as new attitudes, you will empower yourself over food and how you stay in balance with it.

Decide today to accept these ideas and get them working for you.

PRACTICE - Getting New Attitudes

At this point, stop. It's time to take some new attitudes seriously.

New attitudes can come easily if you let them. You're reading the book probably because you need help with food and issues with food. Attitudes are about 80% of the game here—if you can change your view of food, much of the rest of the CAMP system will come readily to you.

Give yourself at least a week to review, contemplate, and accept the Ten Principles before going on to the next chapter. (I know you're eager to get on with the program, but this is important work here!)

Summary of Action steps

1.   Continue writing in your Journal. You are recording your foods each day and some idea of how much you're eating. Keep up that work.

2.   You're also noticing who or what you're blaming for your eating problems. As time goes on, you should be finger-pointing less and less and realizing that you are in control. As changes occur in your outlook, write that in your Journal also.

3.   Starting now, begin reviewing the Ten Principles, *at least once each day.* To help you do this, reserve a page in your Journal (the very last page is good for this) and copy the statements of the Ten Principles there. Then, each day as you write in your Journal, review the Principles and keep them in your mind.

4.   Jot down in your Journal how you could bring the Principles into your life. If each of the Principles is true, what does that mean to you? If you truly believed each Principle, how would it change your approach to food? Put your thoughts down and keep the Principles in the forefront of your awareness.

Progress

At this point in the CAMP system you are:

❏   Continuing your daily food Journal.

❏   Continuing to evaluate to whom or to what you're giving up power over food and seeing yourself each day on the Food Economy diagram.

❏   Reviewing the ten CAMP Principles every day, recording in your Journal any ideas or insights that come to you about the principles and how they relate to your eating.

7.

Mindful Eating: Arriving

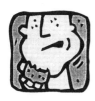 The longer I live the more I am convinced that most of us sleepwalk through large portions of our lives. We go through the activities of each normal day completely unaware of what is really going on around us. Instead of paying attention to the present moment, we allow our minds to dwell in the past, endlessly living over and over the regrets and glories of our histories, or we fantasize about the future and whatever it might bring. We worry about things over which we have no control. We dream impossible dreams and then ponder why they don't come true. And we fill our minds with judgements and opinions about other people, objects, events and even ourselves.

Meanwhile, the old Earth keeps a-turnin' and we miss it all—the sights, sounds, smells and tastes of the world. The old adage that we should "stop and smell the roses" seems simple enough, and we all know about it, but for some reason it's so difficult to do consistently.

Most of us give very little thought to the food that we eat. We approach food mindlessly, and we eat it mindlessly. After we have eaten, we have only a vague recollection at best of what the meal was like. Few of us indeed could remember what we ate last week (or even yesterday!).

Food for the Id

The real problem with eating mindlessly is that we turn much of our power over to our subconscious mind, especially the pleasure center of our brain. When we pay little attention to the food we eat, our brain says, "Hey, this stuff is great. How about some more!" Food is plentiful and easy to get, so we listen to the brain and pile on more food. All of this happens at the very edge of our awareness, until one day we can't get our pants fastened or our skirt zipped, and we wonder why.

Clearly, the mindless approach to eating is no way to honor the great gift of food. What is needed here is a different approach—one that forces us (finally) to pay attention to our food and what it means to us in our lives. That new approach involves *mindfulness*.

What is Mindfulness?

Mindfulness is, quite simply, a moment-by-moment awareness of things.

With mindfulness, we pay attention to what is going on around us. We crank up our awareness and notice all the details. We stop and smell the roses, noticing their color, aroma, shape, size, and yes, even their thorns.

With mindfulness, we wake up from the half sleep in which we normally live. We are alert, responsive, attentive. Aware of all the distractions from outside sources and from our own minds, we instead concentrate on what is happening right now, where we are. This sounds easy, but it can be difficult. As human beings, we have built-in mechanisms that allow us to operate on auto pilot.

Few of us can remember learning to walk, but if you've ever watched an infant struggle with walking you can imagine what your own effort was like. At first, every step is a disaster and a monument to imbalance. Later, the steps become more confident, but we have to concentrate on every aspect of the step: where we place our feet, what muscles to relax or tighten, when to lift each leg, etc. Through practice and over the weeks and months, however, the steps become better and better until one day we don't even have to think about them any more. And that makes sense—life is tough enough without having to think about every step.

The brain is wired to handle routine tasks without much thought. Unfortunately, that applies to eating as well, and that's where we can get into difficulties.

With mindfulness, our actions are deliberate. I like the phrase that mindfulness is "living life on purpose." We act consciously, with intention. Out actions are careful, slow, premeditated.

With mindfulness, we can find a way to live our lives with more dignity, grace and honor. We cherish moments more, find peace in the simplest acts and spend more time in the present moment, the only moment we really have.

As simple as all this sounds, being mindful on a continuing basis is very difficult for most people, at least at first. With practice, though, mindfulness does become easier. Given enough practice, mindfulness can become as natural as breathing (something else we do without any thought!).

Mindful Driving

If you were to drive a car mindfully, you would be aware of all aspects of your driving. You would pay attention to the feel of your hands on the steering wheel. You would notice the tension in your ankle as your foot rested on the gas pedal. Each bump in the road would receive your attention. All of the sights around you—the other cars, houses, mailboxes, clouds, everything—would be of endless fascination. All the images, sounds, odors and vibrations of the experience would be your world as you drove, and your mind would be fully present in each moment during the entire trip.

Compare that to the way most of us drive each day to work. We sit trance-like behind the wheel, our eyes glazed over as we think about the day ahead, our responsibilities, the argument we had the night before, the co-worker we hate working with, what we'll do "one day" when we finally win the lottery, and so forth. It is only when we finally arrive at work that we realize we have absolutely no memory of how we got there or what happened during the drive.

Sadly, we live most of our lives "asleep at the wheel," little aware of what is going on during the present moment. And when we step out of the present moment, we lose—forever—those moments of our lives. It's as if we weren't alive during those times at all.

In the Spotlight

One way to understand mindfulness is to imagine your consciousness as a spotlight. The spotlight represents where your mind *really* is at any given moment.

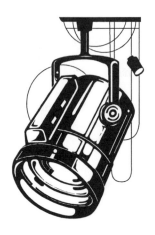

When you brush your teeth in the morning, your spotlight of your consciousness may be, at least at first, on the toothbrush as you put toothpaste on it. Then, you begin brushing, and the spotlight moves into your mouth as you notice the feel of the brush, the taste of the toothpaste, the sound of your brushing. Soon, however, the spotlight moves on—now you're thinking about the day ahead and how you will get everything in. During this time, your spotlight is shining on the future as you imagine it.

Perhaps next you comb your hair. The spotlight shifts to your head, but only for a moment. Then, you're off thinking about the checks that you have to write today.

All day long, in fact, your spotlight moves and flits, shining here and there. Sometimes it's in the present. Often, it's in the past or future, shining on some problem, concern, fantasy, worry or idle thought. Through all of this, you have the rather remarkable ability to bring your spotlight back to the present for just a second every once in a while— *that's* how you can drive to work and get there safely but never remember a thing about it.

During meals, our spotlights shine far and away. Rarely do we bring our spotlights to rest on the food itself, genuinely turning our attention to it.

The CAMP system, however, brings mindfulness to front-and-center stage. As the "M" in CAMP, mindfulness in general, and mindful eating in particular, play a huge role in changing the way we approach, enjoy, honor and relate to food. Mindful eating is the second path to personal control and power over food.

Four Aspects of Mindful Eating

Mindfulness in the CAMP System involves four types of awareness:

- Arriving
- Awakening
- Tuning In
- Service

The rest of this chapter deals with **Arriving**. Here you will learn how to arrive at a meal and to simply become aware of the food in your mouth.

Chapter 8 develops ideas about **Awakening** to food and all its characteristics. In this chapter you'll learn to pay attention to many aspects of food and the effort to bring it to your table or hands.

Chapter 9 covers the concept of **Tuning In** to what your body tells you before, during and after you eat.

Chapter 10 looks into mindfulness as **Service**—all the activities that surround and support your eating.

Arriving

Arriving at a meal refers to mindfully *approaching* food. Before eating, we take a moment to become aware of the food we are about to consume. We give ourselves reminders of what tasks we have to do, how we are going to eat the food, and why we are eating to begin with.

Wake Up!

Any time that food enters your personal, it is time to pause and say to yourself: "Wake up! This is food. Wonderful but dangerous stuff. Handle with care. Be mindful with every step. I have work to do! I can't take it for granted any more."

Setting aside a moment of arrival at each meal gives you the chance to say these kinds of comments to yourself. You remind yourself of the work ahead. You set an intent that you will eat the food with respect both for it and for yourself. You will regard the misuse of food as a risky activity, full of peril and liabilities. Your arrival time also lets you think about how you're in control, that you can make the decisions about what you're going to eat and how much.

Over and over I hear from students: "The CAMP system is a great program and makes a lot of sense; the problem is that I forget to do it!"

I tell them: you must learn to *arrive* at your food.

Strategies

Here are a few simple, effective strategies to help you *arrive* at food:

- Centering breaths
- Body action
- Centering sound
- Smelling the food
- Visual cues
- Centering words

Centering Breaths - Using the breath to center yourself can be amazingly powerful. It's also convenient—the breath is with you all the time, available to use in this way.

Anytime before you begin eating, take four silent but deep breaths. While you're breathing, think about the food that you're going to eat. Imagine yourself eating the food. Calm yourself and notice the food carefully. Bring yourself fully into the present and remind yourself that you have work to do ahead as you eat.

Body Action - Any movement of the body can serve as a wake-up ritual that gets your mind in the present. You could fold your hands, snap your fingers (quietly), touch your ear, tap your palm, or any other action that would mean to pay attention to the food. Find an action that works for you and that reminds you to pay attention. Use it each time you eat. Develop a habit and invite mindfulness to your meal.

Centering Sound - Sounds are powerful reminders of getting to work and waking up around food. A small bell at the table is a wonderful start. Ring the bell and let it ring until the sound is completely gone. During the time the bell is ringing, think about the food and imagine yourself eating it. You could also strike a small meditation bowl or a chime. One family that attended my class plucked a harp string at the start of the meal. Be creative!

Smelling the food - Almost all foods have odors. These chemicals, known as volatiles, are detected in your nose as aromas. Paying attention to the smell of your food at the beginning of a meal can help you arrive. (Actually, it's a good idea to frequently smell your food. When your brain detects these volatiles, it thinks it's eating. So the more you smell your food the more the brain is satisfied that you're getting nourishment.)

When you first encounter food, deliberately notice its aromas. If you're eating alone, get your nose right down next to your foods and take a good whiff. Let the smells be your wake-up call to pay attention to the food and the tasks you have ahead.

Visual cues - A sign or other visual cue can be a powerful wake-up call. Place an object on your table that will remind you to arrive at your meal. It's best to select an object that has meaning to you and that you wouldn't usually see at the table. I give some of my clients small, smooth stones to put next to their plates. The sight of the reminds them to bring attention to the meal.

You could also place a brightly-colored cloth over your plate or silverware. Before you eat, you have to remove the cloth. The sight of the cloth and the action of removing it are clear reminders to arrive at the meal.

Centering words - Reciting specific words before eating can be a very important way to pause, give thanks and bring your attention to the food. You might say to yourself (or out loud) the names of the foods you see or the names of the plants and animals that contributed to your meal (e.g., "hamburger…bread…. salad….cow… wheat…cucumber…lettuce... apple….sugar cane.")

Before CAMP, I never considered why many cultures and religions say a grace. Why be thankful for food and not other things? Why not say thanks for the furniture before sitting down or say thanks for the shower before taking one? The answer has to do with the great value of food, its gifts and the effort to produce it. In cultures where food was scarce and obtained through great struggle, it just made sense to pause and express appreciation. In today's fast-paced society, such a practice has fallen out of favor with many. It's time to revive it!

You might use a standard grace or poem, or make one up. Here is a simple grace that I've given to my students and clients:

The CAMPer's Grace

*May I accept this food with deepest gratitude,
mindful of the many sacrifices and efforts to bring
it here today.*

*May I honor this food by taking only what I need,
by putting it to use to the greater good, and by
eating it with attention and appreciation.*

*And by honoring this food, may I honor myself as I
strive to live in dignity and grace and live my life in
a more sacred way.*

Arriving at food is the essential first step to mindful eating. It is the grounding on which all other stages of mindful eating rest. The "Practice" below will get you started on arriving. Do this exercise for least three days, and beyond that continue your arriving as part of your new and permanent way of eating.

PRACTICE - Arriving at Food

Arriving at food is a life-long change in your eating, and success will hinge on finding the right way to arrive. Over the next three days (and beyond), make a deliberate effort to explore arriving at your food, whether in meals or snacks.

Find one or more of these strategies (covered in this chapter) with which you're comfortable and begin using them with each encounter with food.

- Centering breaths
- Body action
- Centering sound
- Smelling the food
- Visual cues
- Centering words

Or, develop your own strategies.

The lesson from my CAMP students and clients is that most people have the most difficulty *remembering to arrive at food*. Take the next three days to get it right, so you won't have to struggle with this part of the CAMP system.

The idea here is to think of food—any kind of food—as wonderful but dangerous if mishandled. Any time you come into contact with food, remind yourself to wake up, that there is serious work ahead just paying attention to the food.

Progress

At this point in the CAMP system you are:

❑ Continuing your daily food Journal.

❑ Continuing to evaluate to whom or to what you're giving up power over food and seeing yourself daily on the Food Economy diagram.

❑ Reviewing the ten CAMP Principles every day.

❑ Selecting one or more strategies for arriving at food and using those strategies with every meal. Record in your Journal what works, what doesn't, and the difference the strategy has made in your eating.

8.

Mindful Eating: Awakening

In the last chapter, we learned of the importance of *arriving* at food.

When we arrive, we open ourselves up to genuinely experiencing our food. We invite ourselves to pay attention to what we eat and how our bodies respond.

Once we have arrived, the next stage in mindfulness is Awakening. Here, we direct our attention to all the aspects that food has to offer.

Waking up to food means that we purposefully give our attention to the food as we eat it. With mindful eating, you are aware of *every bite* you take.

- You pay attention to *each bite*.
- You chew the food slowly and thoroughly before you swallow it.
- You think about the food: how it tastes, how it feels, its texture, its temperature, its mixture of flavors and aromas.
- You allow your mind to even consider where the food came from, how it grew and how it will soon become a part of you.
- In short, you fully awaken to your meal *and to each bite*.

Only when each bite is completely chewed (and you've enjoyed every bit of it) do you swallow. You swallow slowly and thoughtfully, allowing the food to pass over the taste buds throughout your mouth.

This is a new way of eating to most people. Few of us even bother to think about the mouthful of food we're working on. We're too involved in our thought, conversation, schedule or entertainment to give food any thought. And if we are thinking about food, we're thinking about the *next* bite or perhaps about finishing quickly to get to the dessert or out the door.

On the other hand, the awakened eater takes his or her time with food. Eat bite has its moment of attention. The act of eating slows down, becomes more thoughtful, deliberate, honorable. We honor food for its gifts, recognizing that the food feeds our bodies, minds and spirits.

Back to the Spotlight

In the last chapter, we described the human consciousness as a spotlight. Wherever your spotlight falls is where your attention is. When we awaken to food, we control the spotlight and place it on each bite of food. This takes practice, persistence and discipline. Many other activities and requirements fight for our time and attention during the day. Slowly, we can learn to control the spotlight, to bring it to the food as we eat each bite.

Silverware Down!

Just for fun, the next time you're in a restaurant carefully observe how other people are eating. Notice how they load up a fork, put a wad of food in their mouths and, while still chewing away, they're loading up the fork for the next bite. It's obvious that they're not thinking at all about the food in their mouths no matter how delicious it might be. In fact, they're probably not thinking about food at all.

When we turn our attention to the *next* bite, we miss completely the food we're eating. Instead of *enjoying* the food we're chewing, we allow

ourselves to focus on matters beyond the present moment. This is
mindless eating, and with it we spin out of balance with food.

As a CAMPer eating *mindfully*, however, you put your fork or spoon
down on the table during the time you're chewing. You give your
attention to the food. Until you're completely finished with what's in
your mouth, you don't spend time loading your fork up with more food.
If you're eating "finger food," such as sandwiches or fried chicken, you
put the food down between bites. If you're eating on the run, you do your
best to *not* take a bite until the food in your mouth is completely chewed
and swallowed. As a mindful eater, you concentrate only on the food in
your mouth.

Mindful eating doesn't mean that you have to eat with your eyes glazed
over, totally out of the conversation or whatever else is going on. You
can learn to eat mindfully and still enjoy conversation, the TV or the
newspaper. But you will have to practice.

The Goal: One Second

In the CAMP system, your goal is to spend at least *one second* during each
bite carefully thinking about your food. For that second, bring your mind
into the present moment, fully concentrating on the food. Then, allow
your mind to go back to whatever else it was doing-conversation, TV,
newspaper, thinking. On the next bite, bring the spotlight back onto your
food for one second. Keep the spotlight there for the full second, and
then allow it to swing away.

Master of the Dancing Light

Over time, you will get better and better at bringing your mind to your
food. At first, it will be work and will require lots of practice. As you
increase your skills, you will find yourself automatically eating this way.
But you must practice to get there and use every encounter with food as
training for your mindfulness skills.

Your goal here is to master the dancing spotlight. You are in control of what you are thinking about. You bring that spotlight to your mouth with every bite, and you make the decision when to let it swing back to other issues. Your spotlight will dance from here to there, once in your mouth during each bite. It is that dance of the light you want to control.

PRACTICE - A Simple Strategy

This chapter will develop many strategies for eating mindfully, being wide awake and aware of your food. A *simple* strategy, however, is a good place to begin, so here's a relatively simple one.

For the next three meals you eat, try this: with each bite, say to yourself, "I have food in my mouth" or "I've just taken a bite." That's all. You don't have to think about anything else or keep you mind on your food for any longer than that. Each bite, you bring the spotlight to your mouth simply to notice that food is there.

If you've taken some bites without remembering to notice them, that's okay. Be gentle with yourself. Merely becoming aware that you failed to notice the food is a big step. Bring your mind back to your food on the next bite, and continue practicing. Over time, you will come to notice your food automatically with each bite. Remember, the CAMP system is a skill that takes weeks and months-start with baby steps to slowly change your eating over time.

What Do I Think About?

As you eat and force your spotlight on your food for once second during each bite, here are just a *few* of the things you can consider:

- the taste of the food
- the texture of the food
- the appearance of the food (colors, patterns, etc.)
- the odors of the food
- its smoothness
- its crunchiness
- its creaminess
- its chewiness

- its juiciness
- its mix of flavors
- its aftertastes
- what plants or animals contributed to the food
- what sacrifices those plants and animals made
- where the food was produced
- what human effort was required to grow, prepare, package, transport and market the food
- the natural resources needed to grow the food
- what gifts the food offers
- how you might receive those gifts
- how you might honor yourself as you put those gifts to use

Clearly, thinking about food can be a life-long activity! You may want to do some research about the foods you eat to see what ingredients they contain or how much effort did it take to raise or produce the foods. An excellent place to start is with food labels. Read about all the ingredients in your foods, clear to the ends of the lists. If you learn that your food contains vinegar, see if you can taste the apples in the food. If the food had corn syrup in it, include thoughts of the corn plants in your mindful reflections.

There is virtually no end to the richness of what you can think about as you eat the food. I encourage my students to bite into an orange and taste the warmth of the sun that shone on it, or to detect the sweat of the person who picked it. Your imagination is the only limit.

A good time to plan what you'll think about is during your "arriving at the food" time. You can decide then all the ways that you'll think about your food. If you have carrots on your plate, you might plan to notice their crunch, their sweetness, their mouth feel, their ultimate sacrifice (since what you eat of the carrot is the root, the plant must die before you can eat it). If you're going to eat steak, you might decide to notice its flavor, its texture, its chewiness, the effort of the cow to produce the muscle tissue, the sacrifice it made for you (like the carrot, it too had to die before you could eat it.)

Every meal, every snack, every bite, your mind is learning to think about the food for one second. Slowly, you gain appreciation for your food and you receive a sense of the great gifts it brings you. It won't matter if you're at the dining room table or munching on popcorn in the movie theater. You become a master of the dancing light, bringing your mind back to the food for each second to think about some aspect of it.

A Chewy Strategy

Mindful eating isn't easy; if it were, we would have probably discovered it early in our lives and we'd be old pros at it by now.

One way to help you remember to eat this way is to count your chewing. I have found that 15 or 20 chews are usually enough to chew up a mouthful of food. If you find your mind wandering and you need something to bring it back with each bite, count your chews. You might decide to chew everything a certain number of times, or simply count the number of chews it takes to get your food ready to swallow.

Mindfulness With Beverages Too

Mindfulness isn't just about the food we eat. We can extend the same care and attentiveness to the beverages we drink. When you take a drink of any beverage, notice its color, taste and flavors. Think about the effort to produce it, to bring it to your table or to your mouth. Each beverage, like each food, is a gift and deserves your attention.

At this point, it's time for a serious practice session. The Raisin Encounter, below, will give you many ideas for mindful eating. As you work through this practice, notice all the ways there are to be mindful. Use this encounter as a model for eating all the other foods you choose.

PRACTICE - The Raisin Encounter

This exercise uses raisins to give you ideas about eating mindfully. To do this exercise, you'll need to get a box of raisins and find some quiet time (maybe 10 or 15 minutes) to devote eating them. When you're ready, continue with the directions below.

1. First, let's just spend a minute looking at the box. We arrive. Consider the effort to make the box, the paper used, the inks, the design. All were expenditures of resources, time and energy.

2. Consider also the transportation of these raisins, the people who handled them in the store, who stocked them on the shelf. More energy, time, effort.

3. Feel the weight of the box in your hand. The weight you feel is largely a factor of the water still in the raisins. Think about the contents and how they are now interacting with you.

4. Open the box, but don't take any raisins out just yet. Look in the box and see the collection of raisins there.

5. Smell the open box. Enjoy the smell of the raisins. Then, enjoy the experience of just smelling raisins.

6. Notice collective color and appearance of the raisins.

7. Remove a single raisin from the box. Set the box aside. Don't put the raisin in your mouth yet. Look carefully at this raisin.

8. Notice its color, its shape, its surface appearance. Feel its texture.

9. Consider what this raisin is. Somewhere, weeks ago, this was a grape on a vine far away. See your raisin as that grape. Imagine the vineyard. Today, this is your raisin. It's in your hand now.

10. Think about how many weeks that grape grew, flourished and ripened.

11. Smell the raisin. Can you detect any odor from a single raisin?

12. To smell the raisin, you had to raise it to you nose. Were you aware of all the muscles it took just to get the raisin to your nose? Part of mindfulness is tuning in to all aspects of the body. In the next step you'll place the raisin in your mouth. As you do, be aware of the motion of your hand and arm. Notice how you can get the raisin in your mouth without even seeing your mouth. Tune in to all your systems and how they work together.

13. Now, put the raisin on your tongue. Don't chew yet. Just feel the raisin on your tongue. Notice how it feels there. Can you tell its size, its shape, or its texture with your tongue?

14. Notice if you can taste anything. Is it fruity? sweet? bitter?

15. Move the raisin around your mouth. Does the raisin feel any different in various parts of your mouth? Can you detect any other tastes as you move the raisin? Become aware of the movements of your tongue and how you can control it.

16. Leave the raisin in your mouth unchewed for a little longer. Is its shape changing? Can you detect that the raisin is expanding as it takes in moisture?

17. Now, begin chewing the raisin. Chew it slowly and carefully. Think about the tastes that are being released. How is the texture changing? (Don't swallow yet-keep chewing slowly.) Spread the chewed raisin all around your mouth. Feel the action of your jaw and the sensation of food on your teeth. Notice how different parts of your mouth may taste different aspects of the raisin.

How would you describe its taste? Sweet? bitter? fruity? grapey? Sense the gift of energy you've received in this raisin.

18. Now, you're ready to swallow. Swallow slowly and gently. Let the raisin go easily down your esophagus. Can you feel it? Follow the food down to your stomach? Can you feel it?

19. Shift your focus back to your mouth and notice any aftertastes? Swallow again and keep the spotlight in your mouth? Do you sense a shift in the taste?

20. Lastly, adopt an attitude of thanks to the raisin, to the grape plant, to all the people that helped bring that particular raisin to you today.

21. Take another raisin and eat it with the same mindful approach. This time, be creative and find other things to think about as you eat it. Take your time and enjoy the raisin. When you're done, put the box of raisins away; they have served their purpose well, and you don't need any more of them right now.

This book provides a number of other practice encounters with food, but the Raisin Encounter is the simplest. Return to it anytime you need a refresher in mindful eating.

This next practice below is your <u>main assignment</u> from this chapter. Follow this procedure for all your meals, snacks, etc.

PRACTICE - Awakening to Food

Starting with your next meal, you will begin to pay close attention to your eating and to the food.

You don't have to put you mind on the food all the time. You may talk, watch TV, read or do whatever you normally do during eating. But from now on, you will devote *one second* during each mouthful to thinking about the food and bringing your spotlight on the food.

Summary of Action steps

1. Every time you encounter food, remember to arrive (see chapter 7) at the food. Find some action that helps you wake up to the food. This action should remind you of the work you have ahead. Indeed, balanced eating takes work-energy, commitment and perseverance.

2. For one second during each bite, focus your attention on the food in your mouth. During the first few days you try this, start simply. Be satisfied with just being aware that there is food in your mouth or that you've taken a bite. For each bite, say to yourself, "I've just put food in my mouth" or "I'm aware of the food in my mouth." That alone will be a great step forward.

   Later on, as you get used to eating this way, begin thinking about the food and its appearance, texture, taste, flavor, chew factors, mouth feel, effort to produce it, sacrifice, etc. You will control your spotlight of consciousness, bringing it into your mouth for a second during each bite.

3. Treat all foods the same: meals, snacks, nibbles, bites, beverages and tidbits. All will be consumed mindfully.

4. To help bring your mind to the food, count the number of chews for each bite. Usually, 15 to 20 chews will be enough to thoroughly chew the food. Count more or less as needed. Use this counting strategy especially if you find it hard to control your spotlight with every bite.

5. As you chew, put your silverware down—no loading up the fork with more food as you chew!

6. Eat slowly and deliberately. Pay attention. Wake up!

7. Chew your food thoroughly before you swallow.

8. One time each week, find a quiet time to eat a small snack or meal completely mindfully. This could be as simple as a few cookies and a cup of tea. During this snack, no TV. No reading. No conversation. Just you and the food. Bring your mind to the eating for the entire time. This is not easy, so be gentle with yourself with this and try it a number of times. As you practice, you will get better.

9. Continue your Journal. Jot down your feelings, observations, and experiences with mindful eating in addition to the regular practice of listing the foods you eat each day.

10. Review the Raisin Encounter often to remind yourself of the many ways you can approach food.

11. Continue to review the Ten Principles of the CAMP system.

Mindfulness is not easy to do, especially if you haven't been trained in it. Most people require lots of practice to get mindfulness going, particularly in stressful or busy situations. The five practice exercises that follow can help you get used to mindful eating and mindfulness in general.

Practice: Mindful Six-cracker Snack

This is a good exercise to come back to from time to time to refresh your approach to food.

For this practice, you'll need six crackers. You could also use six potato chips or six pretzels. Select a food that is relatively simple and easy to eat.

You'll also need some water or tea.

Find a time when you can be quiet for about 10 minutes. Get the crackers and your beverage and, if possible, find a place where you won't be disturbed. Don't bring along any magazines or books. Leave the radio or TV off. For the next few minutes, it's just you, the food and your mindfulness.

As you get quiet, take a moment and just look at the food. Arrive. Be in the present moment and honor the food you're about to eat. Remember CAMP Principles #2 and #3:

> #2 Food is for nourishment-sustenance for body, mind and spirit.
> #3 All food is special and merits our deepest respect-it is a great gift of energy and effort.

1. Place cracker #1 in your mouth. Wake up! As you chew it slowly, notice all the tastes and flavors. Thoroughly enjoy the cracker. Chew it completely. Pay attention to the cracker's saltiness, sweetness and any changes in flavors as you chew it. No hurry here. You have all the time you need to enjoy this one cracker. When you've completely chewed the cracker, swallow it slowly. Then, pause and pay attention to the aftertastes.

2. Before the next cracker, take a sip of water or tea. Just a sip, but pay attention to the liquid and its tastes or temperature, its smoothness and its refreshing effect on your mouth.

3. Place cracker #2 in your mouth. Wake up! This time, notice the crunch and sounds of the cracker as you chew it. How do the sounds change as you chew? What new sounds arise? Take your time and enjoy the moment of listening to your food. Chew completely and swallow.

4. Take a sip of water or tea.

5. Place cracker #3 in your mouth. Wake up! This time, pay attention to how the cracker feels in your mouth. Begin chewing, but for this cracker chew at ½ the normal rate. Notice how the cracker goes from crispy to almost like a liquid. Keep chewing and focusing your mind on the feel of the cracker changing in your mouth. Chew completely and swallow.

6. Take a sip of water or tea.

7. Place cracker #4 in your mouth. Wake up! Begin chewing and center your mind on the texture and edges. Can you use you tongue to feel the shape and surface texture of the cracker? Are the edges sharp or rounded? How do they change as you chew? How do different parts of your mouth react to the texture of the cracker? Chew completely and with great deliberateness-chew on purpose! Swallow.

8. Take a sip of water or tea.

9. Place cracker #5 in your mouth. Wake up! This time, focus on the human effort to make the cracker and bring it to you this day. As you chew, think of all the people who may have been involved. Think of the laborers who picked the plant, the baker, the trucker and the grocer. Consider the person who designed the package and the person who placed in on the shelf in the market. Cultivate a sense of thanks for all the efforts involved. Chew completely and swallow.

10. Take a sip of water or tea.

11. Place the final cracker in your mouth and, while you chew, think about the larger web of activity that produced the cracker. Can you taste the wheat plant or the potato plant or the corn plant? Some of the water in your food came from rains or irrigation; can you sense the cycle of water in your food? Picture the ocean and see the water rising up in evaporation and then falling as rain on the plant that made your cracker. The sun shone on the plant as it grew; taste the sunlight and its energy. The cracker you're eating now is the result of thousands of events and interactions. Feel and taste them all. Chew with care and honor the food you're eating. Swallow.

12. Have another sip of water or tea.

Before leaving this practice, take a moment of thanks and reflect on the wonder of a simple meal with of simple food and how it can feed body, mind and spirit.

The next four practices came about because of requests from my students. "Give us more experience," they said, "in dealing with food in distracting or social situations. It's difficult at parties or other gatherings to be eating and carry on conversations." In these exercises, you will be placing yourself in situations where your attention will be divided. The more you can practice under these kinds of circumstances, the better your mindfulness skills with be.

PRACTICE - Eating and Reading

For this exercise, you will need:

- Some food. Select a simple food such as grapes or crackers. You want to have bite-sized food that's easy to prepare. Popcorn or dry cereal would work.
- A book or a magazine that you haven't read before.
- A quiet place.

1. Begin reading the story or article to yourself.
2. As you read, start eating. Eat slowly, a small bite at a time. Don't hurry.
3. Pay attention to the story, but also force yourself to pay attention to the food for one second during each bite. Think about the taste, flavor, texture, crunchiness, smoothness, sacrifice, effort, etc.
4. Continue reading, following the story, but also pay attention to the food. Do this for five minutes.
5. Don't forget to record this food in your Journal.

PRACTICE - Eating and Television

For this exercise, you will need:

- Some food. Select a simple food, such as grapes or crackers. You want to have bite-sized food that's easy to prepare. Popcorn or dry cereal would work.
- A TV tuned to a show or video you haven't seen before.

1. Begin watching the TV show or video.
2. As you watch, start eating. Eat slowly, a small bite at a time. Don't hurry.
3. Pay attention to the story, but also force yourself to pay attention to the food for one second during each bite. Think about the taste, flavor, texture, crunchiness, smoothness, sacrifice, effort, etc.
4. Continue watching, following the story, but also pay attention to the food. Do this for at least five minutes.
5. Don't forget to record this food in your Journal.

This exercise is important, because when we snack and watch TV we usually go on auto-pilot and think very little about our food. In that mode, it gets easy to overeat.

PRACTICE - Eating and Listening

For this exercise, you will need:

- Some food. Select a simple food such as grapes or crackers. You want to have bite-sized food that's easy to prepare. Popcorn or dry cereal would work.
- A friend or acquaintance willing to talk to you for a while.

1. Ask your friend to describe an interest, a hobby or an experience.
2. As you listen to your friend, start eating. Eat slowly, a small bite at a time. Don't hurry.
3. Pay attention to your friend's story, but also force yourself to pay attention to the food for one second during each bite. Think about the taste, flavor, texture, crunchiness, smoothness, sacrifice, effort, etc.
4. Continue listening, following the story, but also pay attention to the food. Do this for at least five minutes.
5. Don't forget to record this food in your Journal.

This exercise will give you experience paying attention to the spoken word and your food in a social setting or just in dinnertime conversation. It is very similar to the next exercise:

PRACTICE - Eating and Speaking

For this exercise, you will need:

- Some food. Select a simple food, such as grapes or crackers. You want to have bite-sized food that's easy to prepare. Popcorn or dry cereal would work.
- A friend or acquaintance willing to listen to you for a while.

1. Tell your friend about an interest, a hobby or an experience of yours.
2. As you speak to your friend, start eating. Eat slowly, a small bite at a time. Don't hurry. You were probably told as a child not to talk and eat and the same time, but this will be good practice for you, so do it!
3. Pay attention to your own words, but also force yourself to pay attention to the food for one second during each bite. Think about the taste, flavor, texture, crunchiness, smoothness, sacrifice, effort, etc.

4. Continue speaking, but also pay attention to the food. Do this for at least five minutes.
5. Don't forget to record this food in your Journal.

This exercise will give you experience paying attention to your food even when you are speaking.

The previous exercises aimed to get you used to mindfulness in setting where you have to split your attention. Most people find it difficult, but don't let difficulty get you down.

The main thing is to get your awareness going with food. If you find it hard to think about your food while you eat, then just concentrate on being aware of the bite in your mouth or just that you have taken a bite.

If you take some bites without mindfulness, be gentle with yourself. Do what you can to be mindful with the next bite.

This is a slow process, and you're taking baby steps. Over time, this will get easier. Remember that I'm asking you to make changes in part of your lifestyle. Most of us don't like changes very much. If you find yourself resisting, that's normal. If you find yourself coming up with reasons why this won't work, ignore them. Just keep agoin'. You've been eating in one way for (probably) a long time-old habits die hard. Just be aware of that and practice, practice, practice.

Continue the practice exercises in this chapter *for at least a week* before going on in this book.

And above all:

Arrive....Be mindful....Chew your food well.....Empty your

hands....Pause after each swallow....Keep your Journal....

Enjoy your food.....Be kind with yourself and treat yourself well.

Progress

At this point in the CAMP system you are:

❑ Continuing your daily food Journal.

❑ Continuing to evaluate to whom or to what you're giving up power over food.

❑ See yourself daily on the Food Economy diagram.

❑ Reviewing the ten CAMP Principles every day.

❑ Arriving at food at every meal.

❑ Eating with mindfulness, care, attentiveness, if only for a second each bite.

❑ Putting your silverware (or any food in your hand) down as you chew.

9.

Mindful Eating: Tuning In

To this point you have learned to arrive at food and to consider all of its characteristics. As a mindful eater, you are paying attention to your food, turning your spotlight on it at least one second during each bite.

To be aware of food, however, is only part of the story.

The ninth Principle of the CAMP system tells us: If we learn to tune in to the body and trust it, it will tell us when we are in balance and harmony with food.

The underlying idea here is that we can rely on ourselves to know what is good for us and when we are in equilibrium with food.

I know what happened when I ignored the signals from the body. I remember well regularly eating huge meals and then wondering why I felt so tired all the time. My body was telling me to take it easy, that all that food was actually dragging me down.

As my waistline got larger and larger, I remember thinking that they weren't making clothes like they used to—my shirts and pants were definitely shrinking in the dryer. I was ignoring the fact that my extra weight was my body's way of telling me that I was out of balance with food.

I used to eat each meal until I felt stuffed. I thought that being stuffed was how I would know to stop eating. I now know that the "stuffed" feeling was my body's way of saying that I was eating way too much food. But back then *I wasn't tuned in.*

Tuning in takes time and practice. It also requires developing some trust and confidence that our inner wisdom will serve us well.

I call this part of mindful eating "tuning in," because it's like a radio tuner. If a radio isn't tuned to a station all we get is noise. But once the radio is tuned properly, the voices and music come through clearly.

If you attempt to listen to your body without being tuned in, you'll get a lot of noise as well. But when you stop and examine your feelings mindfully, the messages begin to emerge, a little at a time, faintly as first, then stronger and clearer.

With tuning in, we heighten our awareness of our bodies. We extend our attention beyond the food and focus on how our bodies feel before we eat, while we eat and after we eat.

With body awareness, some of your mindfulness is directed to yourself. You tune in and become aware of the rich and important messages your body is telling you.

Tuning In Before Eating

Mindful eating can begin long before you ever get to the dinner table or have any encounter with food. Any moment of the day is an opportunity to inspect your systems and see how you feel about food.

A few hours before a meal you may feel hunger. But what exactly is hunger? How do you know when you're hungry? What exactly are the indications or messages you get that you're body is in need of food? Where are *all* the places you experience hunger? Are you really hungry or are you just bored or lonely or sad? How about your energy levels—do they change as your experience being hungry? What events, sights, sounds or smells trigger your hunger?

Practice - Finding your HQ Through the Day

Stop right now and inspect your own HQ (hunger quotient). Your HQ is a number between 1 and 10.

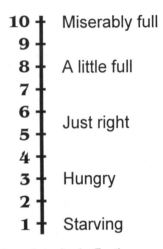

A rating of 1 means that you're completely famished, that all your thoughts are of food and eating, that any minute you're going to start chewing on the carpet, you're so hungry.

A rating of 10 means that you're not hungry at all; you're completely stuffed and you couldn't eat another bite. Many people experience a 10 after the Thanksgiving meal.

How would you rate your HQ right this minute? Find a place in your Journal to write down the time of day and your HQ, a number from 1 to 10. Beside that number write a few words that describe what it's like to have that particular HQ.

10 — Miserably full
9 —
8 — A little full
7 —
6 —
5 — Just right
4 —
3 — Hungry
2 —
1 — Starving

Just deciding on a Hunger Quotient is a big step towards tuning in. For the moment, your mind is in the present and you're mindfully examining yourself. Every time you do this, your sense of self-awareness becomes more keen and more discriminating.

Track your HQ throughout a day. Set up this practice today so you can do it tomorrow.

1. On a blank page in your Journal, create a chart like the one on the right.

2. Starting at 6:00 in the morning (or just before breakfast), record your HQ. (If you schedule is different from the one in the chart, use times that make sense for your daily routine.)

3. Then, every hour on the hour, record your HQ. You may need to carry a small memo pad to jot down your HQs through the day and then put them in the chart later.

4. If you forget to rate your HQ one hour, just go on to the next. The important thing here is to develop a habit of being aware of your body and how it communicates the need—or lack of need—for food.

Time	HQ
6:00 a.m.	
8:00 a.m.	
9:00 a.m.	
10:00 a.m.	
11:00 a.m.	
Noon	
1:00 p.m.	
2:00 p.m.	
3:00 p.m.	
4:00 p.m.	
5:00 p.m.	
6:00 p.m.	
7:00 p.m.	
8:00 p.m.	
9:00 p.m.	
10:00 p.m.	
11:00 p.m.	
Midnight	

5. At the end of the day, look over the trends of your HQ. Did any surprises emerge? Did you feel more in touch with the needs of your body? Did you eat when you weren't really hungry? Record your thoughts in your Journal.

Tuning In While Eating

Many changes occur to our bodies as we eat. Food is being chewed, tasted, swallowed, processed and digested, all at the same time.

That bustle of activity has profound influences on our Hunger Quotient and how we feel about the food. Moment by moment, your system changes in response to the food you're eating, its odors, flavors and quantity.

At this point in the CAMP system, you've been eating each bite of food mindfully (at least for one second), paying attention to the food itself. As we learn to tune in to our bodies, however, we can add new dimensions to our mindful eating: noticing how food, bite by bite, affects our bodies.

When you eat, can you feel the food enter your system after you swallow it? The first bite of a very cold or a very hot food is especially noticeable as it travels down the esophagus into the stomach.

Food affects more of your body than your digestive system. Are you aware of all the muscles involved in eating? While we eat, we can notice the motion of our fingers, hands and arms to get food to our mouths. Did you ever notice that even though you can't see your own mouth, you rarely miss it when you bring food to it? How do we do it?

Chewing food is a complex rhythm of teeth, lips, jaws and tongue. We chew food every day, but we never stop to marvel at the intricate choreography involved in the dance that gets our food ready to swallow. How fast do you chew? What role does your tongue play in getting your food chewed? Do you chew on one side more than the other? When do you move food to one side or another?

When exactly do you stop feeling hungry during a meal? Is it near the beginning? the middle? the end? Does hunger go away quickly or does it subside gently, slowly, a little at a time?

And just how do you decide that you've had enough food? This is an issue we'll explore in some depth in chapter 11, but for now it's worth thinking about. What are the signs that you've had enough food? What is "enough," anyway?

The old measure of "enough" isn't any good anymore. Before, enough meant that all the food was gone. But we've learned from the CAMP principles that it's okay to leave food on our plates. If we're going to get any clues about how much food is enough, we have to tune in and listen to what our bodies are saying.

By tuning in to our bodies while we eat, we gain appreciation of all the dynamics of eating and how those dynamics change throughout a meal.

Practice - Tuning in to Eating

For this practice, you should wait until your HQ is low. In other words, find a time when you're especially hungry. If you have to eat a light breakfast or lunch to be more hungry later on, do it.

It doesn't matter *what* you eat for this exercise, but it will matter that you can count the number of bites you're taking. It may help to have a piece of paper and a pencil so you can tick off the bites as you take them.

Copy the chart on the next page into your Journal. Give yourself plenty of room to write notes.

1. Bring your Journal with the chart you copied to a meal.
2. Before taking any bite of food, record your Hunger Quotient and any notes you feel are important in the first row of your chart.
3. Next, you'll be taking five bites of your meal. Eat each bite slowly, carefully, mindfully, as you've learned to do in earlier chapters.
4. At the end of the fifth bite, go back to the chart. Record you HQ and any notes. Has your HQ gone up? Dropped? How do you feel? Are your cravings for food as strong as they were when you started?

5. Continue the meal, and enjoy bites six through 10. Don't rush, take your time, be deliberate.

6. At the end of the tenth bite, go back to the chart. Record you HQ and any notes. Where are you now?

7. Continue on this way, stopping at bites 15, 20, 25, etc. to record your reactions. When does your HQ rise to 6 or 7 or 8? When are you ready to stop eating? Is it sooner or later than you expected? If you get to bite 50 and you still want more food, continue the exercise and add to your chart until you reach your stopping point.

8. Record this meal in your Journal as usual and add any additional notes about this experience. What have you learned? What do you think would have happened if you had stopped eating before your HQ reached 7 or 8? Did your great hunger at first disappear quickly or slowly as you ate?

After bite #....	HQ	Notes: Tune in and Report
0		
5		
10		
15		
20		
25		
30		
35		
40		
45		
50		

Tuning In After Eating

When you get in the habit of tuning in to your body, the work continues long after your meal is over.

You will continue to digest your food for quite a while after eating. As more and more digested food works its way into your system, your feelings will change. And *what* you ate will determine in no small way how you feel. A meal rich in sugars or other carbohydrates may affect your system quite differently than a meal high in protein and fiber. For me, eating a generous piece of ice cream cake at the office birthday party can get me slumping in a serious way several hours later. (That's not to say that I shouldn't eat ice cream cake, but rather that it's important to pay attention to how foods affect me and when to eat certain foods that keep me feeling well.)

As you develop your internal radio and tune in to your body, here are some things to watch during the hours after eating:

- Is your body happy with the food choices you've made? Notice what you've eaten and how active or tired you are later on. What types of foods give you the most energy hours later? Identify the foods that get you thinking about naptime. Jot down your discoveries in your Journal, and then use what you've learned when you make choices in future meals.

- Is your body happy with the choices you've made about the *amount* of food you're eating? That stuffed feeling is a sign—your body is telling you that you ate too much. How long does that feeling last? Notice how feeling stuffed affects other parts of your life. Take a long, hard look at your food Journal and identify where you could cut back in future meals.

- How does your body feel an hour after eating? two hours? three? four? Few of us have taken the time to learn the landscape of how food affects us and how those feelings change over time. Notice how long your HQ stays high. How many hours after eating does it take for your HQ to drop? When is your HQ the highest?

The questions on this page are important ones for your Journal or for you to answer to yourself. Tuning in to your body—before, during and after eating—will tell you much about how you feel about food and how your body responds to it. For the next two days, explore these questions and find their answers.

Progress

At this point in the CAMP system you are:

❑ Continuing your daily food Journal.

❑ Continuing to evaluate to whom or to what you're giving up power over food and seeing yourself daily on the Food Economy diagram.

❑ Reviewing the ten CAMP Principles every day.

❑ Arriving at food at every meal.

❑ Eating with mindfulness, care, attentiveness, if only for a second each bite.

❑ Putting your silverware (or any food in your hand) down as you chew.

❑ Tuning in to your body, its needs, its enjoyment, it motions and its feelings. You're paying attention to your relationship with food before, during and after meals. Record any and all insights in your Journal.

10.

Mindful Eating: Service

The fourth form of Mindful Eating is an area I call "service." Actually, it's not eating at all. Instead, it's all the things we do that would be considered service *about* food and the act of eating. Just as we can bring our full attention to food as we eat it, we can bring our mindfulness to service about food.

There are three broad categories of service relating to food:

- Food Gathering
- Food Preparation
- Utensil Service

Throughout these categories are many opportunities for us to expand our mindfulness. Every moment that we do, we add to the honor we give to food, and we add dignity and grace to our own lives.

Food Gathering

It wasn't all that long ago that most people had to learn to be self-sufficient. The pioneer spirit that moved our ancestors throughout this county involved a robust knowledge of hunting, fishing, gardening and living off the land.

Today, many of us rely almost exclusively on the corner market to take care of our food needs. We gladly pay others to raise the food, harvest it, package it, transport it and sell it.

Although we may have life jobs and activities that have little to do with getting food, what matters here is not so much *what* we do, but rather *how* we do it.

If you hunt or fish for food, you can do it mindfully. Be aware of the sanctity of life and the great gift of energy and nutrition in the animal you seek.

If you garden or farm, view your work as hallowed, noble, full of honor. See yourself as a steward as you cultivate and harvest plants and their gifts of energy, vitality, texture, taste and aroma.

If we never hunt or fish or garden, though, we can still gather our food mindfully. This requires a bit of rethinking. Shopping for food is usually regarded as an unpleasant necessity, something to get out of the way so we can get on with life. But with mindfulness, every minute is important, every task is significant and every activity can be a chance to stay in the moment.

Practice: Mindful Food Shopping

It may seem strange to bring mindfulness to the supermarket, but what better place to be fully aware of all the choices we have in foods?

Do this practice *every time* you shop. Bring your mind to your task. Honor the food you purchase by realizing how much effort, indeed how much human toil and even sadness, is involved in creating our great food markets.

10. Mindful Eating: Service

1. Arrive at the store by pausing for just a moment. Look around through fresh eyes. See the spectacle before you: aisles and aisles of foods, packages, colors, smells and textures. What a great banquet here. What great gifts of energy and life gathered in one spot.

2. Begin your shopping by keeping your mind in the present. Feel the cart in your hands. See your kids in the cart and sense their presence. Notice the hardness of the floor that you can sense through your shoes. Pay attention to any odors that waft your way. If your cart has a squeaky wheel, make it part of the experience by noticing it.

3. As you look for each item, notice the tremendous variety of choices. Take in all the colors and packages and words and pictures.

4. At the produce section, consider the large sacrifice of the plants, the energy they stored, their efforts to grow. Reflect on what kind of effort it would take if you were to try to grow all those plants.

5. At the meat counter, offer your own thanks to all the animals that died and left behind a legacy of energy and nutrition. Again, reflect on the effort it would take if you tried to raise, slaughter and produce all this food. Contemplate all the other individuals responsible for getting these animal products to you.

6. At the diary counter, imagine the chickens and cows that produced the eggs and milk products. See the dairies. Follow in your mind the farmer who collected the eggs each day or who milked the cows.

7. As you shop, feel your muscles as you reach for objects, hold them and then place them in your cart. Sense the weight, temperature and textures of the objects. Be fully in the moment.

8. Keep up your mindfulness practice as you get to the register. Be aware of each item as you lift it from the cart and place it on the belt. Tune in to the sounds of the moment as items are gathered, lifted, scanned and bagged. Stay in the present. What an amazing thing that you are here at all to experience this! The market is truly a place of infinite richness!

By shopping, you are performing a service to food equivalent to tribal hunting or gathering. This is a crucially important role you play in your life and others. Don't minimize it.

Overeating can begin long before we put food in our mouths. The act of including certain items on a shopping list or deciding to "treat yourself" with each market visit is an act of planning to overeat. Mindfulness in making the shopping list and then in doing the actual shopping can help us out of the habits that lead to overeating.

Any act of gathering food can be an opportunity for mindfulness. A half hour spent in a strawberry patch or in an orchard can be made extraordinary by picking the fruit mindfully, aware moment by moment of the sounds, smells, textures, muscle movements and even the backache. Feel the heat on your back from the sun and the sound of the breeze past your ears. Later on, when you're eating the fruit you picked, recall those golden moments outside as part of your mindful eating.

Food Preparation

If I had to classify the kind of cook I was I'd have to use the phrase "kitchen challenged." Some of the greatest disasters ever produced in any kitchen were by my inept hand. Even so-called "idiot-proof" recipes have been no match for my hopeless lack of skill. If anyone could burn water, I'd be the one. To turn me loose in a kitchen is to condemn it.

And yet, I know that work in the kitchen can be immensely satisfying, and I've enjoyed my attempts at preparing simple foods. Cooking is a way to become intimate with food, its flavors, combinations and nuances. Those who pay careful attention to their work in the kitchen give themselves the opportunity to value and cherish the present moment while giving service to the food.

From start to finish, mindfulness can be used throughout all phases of food preparation.

Selecting a menu can be done with concentration and precision, choosing foods for their nutritional value as well as their other gifts. The next time you sit down to make a shopping list, think of it as a time for mindful reflection.

As you gather the food and your kitchen tools, do so with a great sense of purpose. Keep your mind on the task at hand.

As you cut foods up, blend foods, stir food and all the others actions in the kitchen, stay in the moment. Concentrate on your actions, your intent and the food itself. My wife is a great cook and I watch her in the kitchen sometimes (this is much better than "helping" her in the kitchen as I get myself and the meal in much less trouble that way). She approaches cooking as grand choreography, knowing intuitively how long this dish will take, when to add that liquid, when to start that pan, when to make that sauce. The bell rings and all the food is ready. Amazing. She is one with the task and, for her, working in the kitchen is sacred work.

The next Practice will give you experience fixing a simple food. The lessons here, however, can be extended for any type of kitchen work you may do.

Practice: Mindfulness Soup

In this simple practice, you're going to fix yourself a can of soup. But this is mindfulness soup and you'll fix it in a careful and attentive way.

1. Select the soup you like—it can be any type, but use a can of soup.
2. Assemble the materials you need: the can, a pot, a can opener, a spoon and a bowl. Place all the materials in one place before you begin. Look at them with fresh eyes. Imagine that this is the first time you've ever seen these items. What do you notice? See the colors, the shine, the metal, the paper, the plastic. These are the tools that serve you, the food and your eating.
3. Before handling the food, wash your hands. It's something you've done a thousand times, but not like this. This time, notice every aspect of washing your hands. Keep your mind completely on the task. Observe the feel of the water on your hand. Add soap and sense its smoothness. Watch it foam. Work it well over your hands and feel every movement. Rinse your hands and examine the feeling of soap washing away, the touch of the water and the cooling effect of the air. Dry your hands completely, sensing the texture of the towel and its absorbency.
4. Now, open the can of soup. If possible, don't use an electric can opener. Instead, use one of the manual types, which forces you to invest some muscle energy into opening the can. Squeeze the handle against the lid and feel and hear the lid yield. Turn the crank, slowly, deliberately. Donate your effort to the task. Be aware of every hand motion. Can you feel the muscles in your forearms?
5. Remove the lid when the can is open, and slowly set the lid down. Pay attention to the sound it makes when it touches the table or counter.
6. Bring the can to your nose and smell. How many different foods and spices can you detect? Enjoy the aroma of the soup.
7. Empty the contents of the can into the pot or pan. Take a good look at the soup there. See it afresh. Identify all the ingredients by sight.
8. If the directions call for it, add water to the can and then to your soup. Do these actions with great care, as if they were a holy rite.

9. Turn on the heat, mindfully attending to the motion of your arm and hand.

10. While the soup heats, read the label on the can. Take your time—enjoy this waiting moment. Read over the list of ingredients. With each plant ingredient, imagine it growing in a field. See the plant in your mind's eye. Appreciate the plant's gift now heating before you. With each animal ingredient, see the animal and offer thanks in whatever way you can for its sacrifice.

11. As the soup heats, watch for changes in the soup. See the vapor start to rise. See and hear the bubbles as the soup begins to boil. Take in more of the soup's aroma.

12. When the soup is ready, pour (or ladle) it into your bowl.

13. Before carrying the bowl elsewhere to eat the soup, pause and savor this moment, this present moment. Then, with great purposefulness, carry the bowl to the place where you'll eat the soup mindfully.

Utensil Service

Without plates, cups, glasses and silverware, eating would be a messy enterprise. These are the tools of our meals, and they deserve care and attention.

Although we usually regard most of the tasks as chores, service to the utensils of eating provides many moments for mindfulness. These events of our lives include:

- Setting the Table
- Clearing the Table
- Washing Dishes
- Drying Dishes
- Putting Dishes away

Sounds like fun, doesn't it?

Done mindfully, these tasks take on a new look and feel. We can set the table and be in the moment, truly alive. We can see that work as vital, decent and worthy. Because life is a miracle and our existence fleeting, any part of living that we do with purpose and intent is precious, each moment a treasure. This is the great gift of mindfulness: that in the common ordinary minutes of our days are astonishing jewels of existence, remarkable moments of living.

Practice: Putting Away the Dishes

After the dishes have been washed, the job of putting away dishes has to be done. This is noble work, important work. Approach the task not as an obligation but as a wonderful opportunity to dwell in the present and to honor yet another aspect related to eating. Don't put away the dishes just to get on to something else. Rather, put away the dishes to put away the dishes, fully aware of each moment.

1. As you empty the dish drainer or dishwashing machine, take each item one at a time.

2. Keep you mind fully on that item, its use, its characteristics, its feel.

3. Put each item away slowly, carefully. Place it in the cupboard or in the drawer so carefully you make no sound. (This takes practice and patience!) Be aware of your muscles and your movements. Feel the weight of each item and sense how your body interacts with it. Sense that you're doing sacred work here.

4. If some of the dishes are still wet or damp, dry them slowly and thoroughly with a towel. Savor each moment as you prepare the items for putting away.

5. If your mind wanders to other thoughts, simply bring it back onto the task at hand.

6. Continue on this way until all the dishes are put away.

This is just one of many ways to bring mindfulness to Utensil Service. You could do the same type of practice with Setting the Table, Clearing the Table, Loading the Dishwasher, Washing the Dishes, etc. Experiment and explore and bring mindfulness to *every* aspect of handling your meal utensils.

As you continue your mindfulness activities, you will see how they can be applied to life in a much broader perspective.

For example, when you clean the kitchen, wipe its cabinets, mop its floor and scrub its sink, you add to the way to honor food. And when you do this work mindfully, you elevate the work out of drudgery to something much more noble.

When you brush and floss your teeth, you are taking care of another tool important to eating. And yes, you can do that brushing mindfully, keeping you attention to each moment of the task, tooth by tooth.

At the very broadest perspective, when you go to work you are earning money for, among other things, food. Our professions, no matter what, take on new slants when seen through the lens of mindfulness and purpose.

Indeed, mindfulness can be applied to virtually any venue of your life, giving you the opportunities ahead for endless exploration and growth.

Progress

At this point in the CAMP system you are:

❑ Continuing your daily food Journal.

❑ Continuing to evaluate to whom or to what you're giving up power over food and seeing yourself daily on the Food Economy diagram.

❑ Reviewing the ten CAMP Principles every day.

❑ Arriving at food at every meal.

❑ Eating with mindfulness, care, attentiveness, if only for a second each bite.

❑ Putting your silverware (or any food in your hand) down as you chew.

❑ Tuning in to your body, its needs, its enjoyment, it motions and its feelings.

❑ Bringing mindfulness to getting food, preparing food, setting the table, cleaning up, putting dishes away, etc. All of it is sacred work, and through it all you give honor to the food.

11.

Portions: Challenges

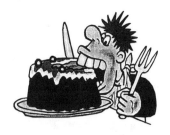

Food portions in this country have gone completely out of control. From our dinner tables to our restaurant tables, the serving sizes are getting bigger and bigger with no end in sight.

Most restaurant "meals" could serve three people nicely. The appetizers alone are enough to fill us up. Then they feed us huge helpings during the main course, and have the audacity to ask if we have room for dessert. Amazingly enough, often we say "yes" and eat it all.

Popcorn in movie theaters now comes in three sizes: Jumbo, Gargantuan and Blue Whale. Getting through even the smallest of these is barely possible.

Buffet restaurants are busy from the time they open to the time they close, full of people filling plate after plate, all attempting to get the best value for their dollar. Bloated and belching, they leave the buffet vowing to eat even more the next time when they return. (I know! I used to be one of them.)

When and where will it stop?

In the CAMP System, the "P" stands for Portions. Managing portions is the third path to personal control and power over food.

Eating too much food has a colossal role in being overweight. Although it's true that people can be overweight from eating inappropriate carbohydrates and fats and other high-energy foods, the main culprit is that most overweight people EAT TOO MUCH. Plain and simple.

Think back to the simple food economy pictured on page 37. We learned there that if we eat more energy than we use, we gain weight. Clearly, if we're going to lose weight we have to eat less food.

That's worth repeating: **Clearly, if we're going to lose weight we have to eat less food.**

But it's tough to do that, in spite of our best intentions. Food is good, abundant and cheap. How do we say "no"?

We have a lifetime of poor eating habits to fight and, for many of us, strong lessons from our childhood to overcome.

Find the Bunny

When I was a little boy, I was often asked to *find the bunny.* No, it wasn't a family pet—it was a drawing on the bottom of my plate. Wanting me to eat well, my parents would encourage me to eat everything on my plate. To give me motivation, they would remind me that the food was covering up a picture of a rabbit. "Find the bunny, Freddy," my mom would say. And when I did, I

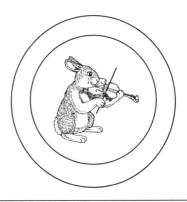

heard "good boy!"

It was a good strategy— perhaps a little too good, as its lessons stayed with me well into adulthood.

Many of my CAMP students report a similar experience with eating. As youngsters, we learned to finish everything on our plates. The old adage "waste not, want not" was driven into our heads.

And as adults we continue to hear our parents' voices from across the years telling us to finish everything on our plates. Dutifully, we obey— older now, we continue to search for the bunny. We give away our power and put on the pounds. Can we undo those powerful lessons learned years ago?

This chapter and the next two chapters will give you new approaches, actions and strategies for making sense of food portions. When you sit down to eat, you will have a plan to determine just how much you *should* be eating and how to sensibly eat to reach that amount.

Once you have established what your portion size is, you'll be able to make wise decisions automatically whenever and wherever you eat. You'll be able to place yourself anywhere you want on the food economy diagram we first studied in chapter 5.

The chapter you're reading now deals with seeing **Portions as Challenges**. You will be asked to challenge just about everything dealing with your eating.

Chapter 12 deals with **Portions as Sensation**. Much of our eating has to do with how good food tastes, and in chapter 12 you'll learn a technique unique to the CAMP system that will help you satisfy food cravings while eating smaller portions.

Chapter 13 looks at **Portions as Boundaries** and includes techniques of setting up your own food boundaries.

The Many Challenges of Portions

Who decides how much you eat during each meal? You may think that you do, but that's too easy an answer. As we've seen, we give power away and let others decide. Your parents decide when they put food on your plate and then tell you to eat it all. The chef decides when he or she puts a "serving" on your plate and gives it to the waiter to bring to your table. The food manufacturer decides by putting only so much food in the box or suggests a serving size on the food label. And on and on. We rely on *others* to determine what's right for us, and many times the people making the decisions don't even know us!

Ever notice the label on a bag of potato chips? How many chips are considered one serving? How many chips are right for you? Some bags proclaim that a serving size is 13 chips. Thirteen chips?! That number may make it easier to compare one snack food to another, but it has little meaning to what your body may need. If you're like most people, you open the bag and eat the chips until you don't want any more. Few of us are counting the chips, but rather let the chips fall where they may.

As you consider portions, you should allow yourself to challenge just about everything you do in relationship to food and the amounts you eat:

1. How much do you eat of each food?
2. How much do you really need of each food?
3. How does the type of food influence how much of it you eat?
4. How big a bite do you take at one time?
5. How long do you chew the bite?
6. At what rate do you chew your food?
7. How long do you wait between each bite?
8. How much do you enjoy each bite?

Whew! That's a lot to consider. And making it more difficult is that these are things that we learned to take for granted long ago. How many of us, for example, ever stop to think about how quickly or slowly we're chewing our food?

The good news is that *you are in control* of all of these relationships. Once you are aware of that, <u>you can decide to take power</u> over how much you're eating and how you're eating it.

1. **You can decide how much you eat of each food.** At a restaurant, you are in control, not the chef. You see the amount of food on your plate as merely a suggestion, not an imperative. No longer do you listen to your parent voice telling you to "find the bunny." You ignore the label on the potato chip bag and eat six or ten or twelve chips, because that's enough for you.

2. **You can decide how much you really *need* of each food.** You've been tuning in the body radio and you're discovering your body's requirements. From CAMP Principle #2, you're learning that food is primarily for nourishment, not for the dozen other uses we put to food.

3. **You can decide how the type of food influences how much of it you eat.** Although all foods are gifts, some foods have more energy than others do. The portions you select are geared to their energy gifts. You may choose to eat a much larger portion of steamed carrots than of chocolate cake, not because carrots are *better* than cake, but because cake has more available energy than carrots, and you're seeking a balance in your own food economy.

4. **You can decide how big a bite you take at one time.** Living a life with more grace and dignity (Principle #10) involves moderation and eating with some elegance. You know what bite size makes sense in your mouth and you choose put the appropriate amount on your fork or spoon.

5. **You can decide how long you chew each bite.** You don't have to swallow your food half-chewed. If you've been eating mindfully up to this point, you're learning to chew your food completely. It's *you* making the decision of when the food is ready to be swallowed. Every bite is a deliberate act.

6. **You can decide how quickly or slowly you chew your food.** It may never have occurred to you that the rate at which you chew is a

choice. We just chew. But you can control it. You can slow it down or speed it up. It's your choice (and your power!).

7. **You can decide how long to wait between each bite.** No need to hurry. The next bite will be there, waiting. Slow down. Enjoy. Make a choice. It is the blackness between the stars that makes them so beautiful. Similarly, it is the pauses between bites that adds to the dignity and grace of our eating.

8. **You can decide how much you allow yourself to enjoy each bite.** Food is there for our enjoyment. Why rush through it? You smell the roses, you notice a beautiful sunset. Why not make the choice to take pleasure in every bite, every morsel, every type of food.

Practice: How Many Potato Chips?

Deciding ahead of time how much food you will eat is a terrific strategy and one I use all the time, especially when I make myself lunch at home. I'll count out how many crackers, how many grapes, how many small pieces of cheese, etc., I'm going to eat, and then I stick to it. I remember how many of each type of food so I can record the amount in my Journal. As the days go by, I can change the numbers as I seek to maintain my balance with food.

For practice, let's eat some potato chips or pretzels or rice cakes. Pick a food that you enjoy. You'll also need a plate or a paper towel and a glass or bottle of water.

1. Find a quiet time—you'll need about 5 minutes.
2. Select the food you wish to eat. Good potato chips are excellent for this practice, because people often find it difficult to stop eating them.
3. Count out 15 chips. Find 15 whole, unbroken chips for this exercise. Place the chips in front of you on the paper towel or on the plate. Put the bag away, out of sight.
4. Before eating any of the chips, arrive at the chips. Think about the gift they represent. Offer thanks to the potato for its energy and its life. Imagine yourself eating the chips and how you'll do it mindfully, carefully, slowly, one chip at a time.
5. Now, place a chip in your mouth and eat it in the CAMP way. Chew thoroughly and swallow only when you're ready. Pause and notice any aftertastes. Enjoy the chip.

6. Ask yourself: "Could I stop here? Am I in control? Is this chip enough?" Notice and tune into what your body is telling you. Note your HQ.

7. Before going on to the next chip, take a small sip of water. This clears the palate and prepares it for the next chip. As you will learn in the next chapter, water will play a crucial role in the CAMP system. This practice will introduce you to using water as a clearing agent.

8. Now take another chip, eating it mindfully, chewing it thoroughly, enjoying it completely. Swallow when you're ready and clear with a sip of water.

9. Continue on this way. Notice along the way any changes in your HQ and if you could stop eating after chip #6 or #9 or maybe #12. Could you leave three chips uneaten? Could you throw the last five or four chips away? (Remember CAMP principle #6 that says It is far better to leave some food uneaten than to eat more than is needed.)

10. If you wish, finish 14 chips. Don't go back for more. Ask yourself if you're satisfied with the 15 chips. Do you really need more? Then, throw the 15th chip away.

11. Record this snack in your Journal and include any reflections about this practice.

12. Try the practice again in a day or so, but this time, count out only 12 chips. Some days later, you could try it again with perhaps eight chips. Could you do this practice with just three chips? Would you enjoy them? Would three be enough? The only way you'll find out—and to learn about yourself and the power you're seizing back—is to explore.

Power over portions is power over food. When you challenge everything about how you *were* eating, you change how you *will* eat.

The practice below can be used any time, with any meal. Try it again and again. We come to control over food by three main paths, and being a master of your food portions is one of those paths.

Practice: You're In Control

During any meal, eat all the food mindfully, making sure to eat at least one bite with each of the items below in mind.

1. Decide how big a bite you'll take. Less food on the fork can still taste as delicious as a full fork. Take a small bite, and make the next one a little smaller. Savor the food regardless of how big the bite is.

2. Decide how fast you're going to chew. Force yourself to chew more slowly. Halfway through the chewing, stop chewing completely for five seconds. Then resume your chewing. On the next bite chew even more slowly. Put yourself in control.

3. Decide how long you're going to chew the food. You normally chew your food completely, but why not a few extra chews? Chew one bite 20 times, the next bite 25 times and the next bite 30 times.

4. Decide that you're going to wait a longer time between bites. Spend the time noticing the aftertastes, engaging in conversation, or simply reflecting on being in the present moment. Don't hurry. The food will still be there when you're ready for the next bite. Wait 5 seconds between bites. Then, wait 10 seconds. Try 15 seconds. Or 20. What's right for you? Are you in control?

5. Decide that you're going to enjoy the food. Even if you're eating something very simple, such as plain rice or unbuttered bread, make up your mind that your going to find pleasure and delight in each bite of it. Take a bite of simple food and say (aloud or to yourself) "Mmmmmm." No matter how simple the food may be, honor it by enjoying it.

6. Record your meal in your Journal as always, along with your impressions of taking your time and focusing in on these control issues. Did you actually feel more in control? Were you aware that you were making your own decisions during this practice about how to eat?

Progress

At this point in the CAMP system you are:

❑ Continuing your daily food Journal.

❑ Continuing to evaluate to whom or to what you're giving up power over food and seeing yourself daily on the Food Economy diagram.

❑ Reviewing the ten CAMP Principles every day.

❑ Arriving at food of every meal.

❑ Eating with mindfulness, care, attentiveness, if only for a second each bite.

❑ Putting your silverware (or any food in your hand) down as you chew.

❑ Tuning in to your body, its needs, its enjoyment, it motions and its feelings.

❏ Bringing mindfulness to getting food, preparing food, setting the table, cleaning up, putting dishes away, etc.

❏ Challenging just about everything to do with how you were eating in the past. You're examining how much you eat, how fast you eat, how you chew, when you stop, etc. You're beginning to control how fast you chew, how many chews you take for each bite and how much you wait between bites.

12.

Portions: Sensation

Pizza is one of my favorite foods, and I can't have it too often. I wouldn't mind if they passed a law saying that we had to eat pizza four times a week.

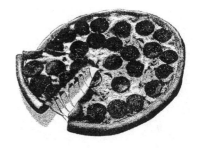

If I know I'm going to have pizza for dinner, I might start thinking about it that morning. I await with great anticipation biting down into that glorious combination of dough and cheese, tomato sauce and pepperoni. As the hours tick by, my craving for pizza grows. Ah, to take that first bite. Truly there is a heaven, and it's round with eight slices.

Finally, dinnertime arrives and the pizza is before me, hot and bubbly and oozing with promise. And indeed, that first bite is a gustatory delight. The second bite is pretty good, too. The third bite is okay. And the fourth bite? Yeah, it's okay. But I wish all the bites could be as good as the first one.

One of the problems some people have with reducing portions is that they feel cheated. They're used to eating a certain amount, and feel somehow robbed if they have to stop eating before they get their usual quantity of food.

I faced this problem myself when I started on my new way of eating. How can I be satisfied with two slices of pizza when I'm used to four (or more!) slices?

One of the solutions is related to craving and the role of sensation in eating. My hunger for pizza is a craving, a mindless, automatic longing for that wonderful food. I seek sensation. I desire the feel and taste of pizza in my mouth. I yearn for that magnificent first bite of pizza, that explosion of pizza taste in my mouth.

But if I'm going to reduce my portions and eat less pizza, is there a way I can extend that feeling of enjoying the experience of the very first bite? Is there a method for extending the wonderful "first bite" experience to the many bites after the first?

The Rule of Four

There is, and the technique that will do it is based on a totally unscientific theory of mine that I call the Rule of Four. The Rule of Four states: Most cravings are satisfied in the first four bites of any food.

If you love steak, notice the next time you eat it that the first four bites are the very best. By the time you reach bite #5, you're still enjoying the steak and it's still delicious, but your cravings for steak have substantially diminished.

Somewhere during the first four bites, the brain is getting the message that the food it craves has arrived and is in abundance. The brain relaxes, and the cravings shrink.

From this idea arises the next CAMP technique. If we can extend the experience of the first four bites, our brains will reach a deeper level of satisfaction and will be happy with less food.

Clearing

The way we keep the fresh experience alive longer is to clear the palate after every bite. We take away the old tastes and set up the mouth to receive the next bite. And the only logical substance that can do this? Water.

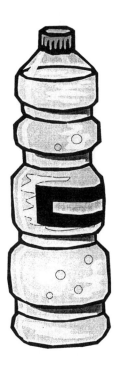

The act of "Clearing" is taking a sip of water after each (and every) bite of food. This sip is just that— a sip, only enough water to bring the mouth back to a clean state. Water is neutral, with no taste or odor of its own. It adds nothing to the flavors of a meal, and goes nicely with everything.

I'm not suggesting that you have to give up your favorite beverages. If you're used to tea or soda or coffee or anything else, by all means continue with those beverages.

But now you'll bring a second liquid to your eating if you're used to another beverage. The water, however, is not a beverage—it is your clearing agent.

Beverages are Foods Too

From this point on, you will be taking a sip of water after all bites of food. You will also be taking a sip of water after each sip of a beverage. In the CAMP system, treat any beverage other than water as a food.

So after each bite of food or drink of a beverage, before you pick up your fork or the iced tea glass again, pause and clear with water.

No matter what you eat, no matter when you eat, include water for clearing.

With clearing, a typical meal might look like this:

bite of chicken
    = clear =
bite of chicken
    = clear =
bite of potato salad
    = clear =
drink of iced tea
    = clear =
bite of chicken
    = clear =
bite of coleslaw
= clear =

and so forth. Notice that you'd clear after each bite and after each drink, now matter what the food or drink was.

A few of my students have told me that they enjoy the flavors of certain foods *combined* with a beverage. They like to take a bite of food and mix it with a sip of their coffee or cola or some other beverage. When I introduced the idea of clearing, these individuals expressed concern that they might feel deprived if they can't mix foods and beverages.

I tell them to enjoy their food! Never be deprived. Simply consider the *mixture* of food and beverage as a single food, and then clear after eating the mixture. Throughout the entire CAMP program, find ways to be creative as you bring CAMP ideas into your own life. For any CAMP problem that comes up, think of "how you could" and not "why you can't."

Other Benefits to Clearing

Clearing has benefits beyond convincing the mind that it's getting fresh new experiences of food and drink.

- Clearing will help you to slow down. The very act of stopping to clear after each bite extends the time you'll be with your food. That extended time helps your brain accept less food as enough food.
- Clearing adds a rhythm to your eating. You can develop a pace and tempo to eating that you otherwise didn't have.
- It enhances the mindfulness in eating. You have yet another deliberate action to do many times during each meal.

And if You Forget?

If you find that you've forgotten to clear, be gentle with yourself. Learning to incorporate clearing in all your eating takes time, willingness, practice and attention. Pick up where you are and begin clearing when you can.

On the other hand, clearing is an essential part of the CAMP system. If you find yourself thinking right now of why you don't need to do this or how impractical this is, it may be time to again evaluate where you want to be in your balance with food. Clearing is a new idea and your mind is suspicious of anything new. Ignore those uncertainties. Decide right now that you're willing to add clearing to your repertoire of CAMP strategies.

With clearing, I can have my two pieces of pizza and feel satisfied. Actually, I enjoy it more, because more of the bites of pizza taste like the first bite at the height of my cravings.

Practice: Popcorn Snack and Clearing

The CAMP system is a way of eating everything, snacks included.

For this exercise, you will need some popcorn, a beverage and some water for clearing.

If you have access to a microwave oven and can pop the corn there, that's best. Otherwise, buy a bag of popcorn at the market.

1. Pop the popcorn or get a bag of popcorn. Get good popcorn, the kind you crave. Before eating the popcorn, throw at least half of the popcorn away. Actually put it in the garbage can. You are going to limit your portions, and less popcorn will now be as satisfying. If it is difficult for you to throw the food away, remember CAMP Principle #6: It is far better to leave some food uneaten than to eat more than is needed.

2. Place the remaining popcorn in a bowl. (If there's still some left over, throw the leftovers away also.)

3. Pour yourself a favorite beverage.

4. Get a glass or bottle of water for clearing.

5. Take the popcorn, your beverage and the water to a place where you can eat the popcorn mindfully.

6. Begin by taking one kernel of popcorn. Chew it slowly, carefully, deliberately. When it's thoroughly chewed, swallow.

7. Clear with a sip of water.

8. Now take a drink of your beverage. Don't hurry. Don't gulp. Enjoy the beverage as a food. Think about where the beverage came from, how it was made, and the effort to get it to you. Swallow.

9. Clear with a sip of water.

10. Next, take one kernel of popcorn. Chew thoroughly. Swallow.

11. Clear

12. You decide (after all, you are in control) whether next to eat more popcorn or take a drink. Whatever you do, be sure to clear afterwards.

13. Continue on, eating one kernel of popcorn at a time, clearing after each or taking sips of your beverage, clearing after each.

14. When you reach the bottom of the bowl ask yourself if that amount of snack was satisfying. Most people do, but if not, that's okay; you will be learning over time to be satisfied with less, and you've thrown the rest away to help you quit at this point.

Clearing will be a new part of your eating, starting with your very next meal. It's a very powerful strategy to help you reduce your portions and has the benefit of increasing your enjoyment of food.

Progress

At this point in the CAMP system you are:

❑ Continuing your daily food Journal.

❑ Continuing to evaluate to whom or to what you're giving up power over food and seeing yourself daily on the Food Economy diagram.

❑ Reviewing the ten CAMP Principles every day.

❑ Arriving at food of every meal.

❑ Eating with mindfulness, care, attentiveness, if only for a second each bite.

❑ Putting your silverware (or any food in your hand) down as you chew.

❑ Tuning in to your body, its needs, its enjoyment, it motions and its feelings.

❑ Bringing mindfulness to getting food, preparing food, setting the table, cleaning up, putting dishes away, etc.

❑ Challenging just about everything to do with how you were eating in the past by becoming aware of how you eat, how fast, how long you pause between bites, etc.

❑ Clearing after every bite with a sip of water. You're treating all solids and liquids are food, and you clear after any bite, slurp, lick or sip.

13.

Portions: Boundaries

We live in an age when boundaries are becoming increasingly indistinct. Generally, our society is one of excess, of "get it now," of "never mind the rules," and of "I like it so I'll do it."

That same mindset has spilled over into the eating arena. We eat food any time, any where, as much as we want and of whatever type we want. No one is there to say "enough" or "careful." And with that our portions have gotten bigger and bigger and bigger.

When I was young, I remember going to a small neighborhood store and reaching into a cooler full of water. Standing in that frigid water were many bottles of soda: grape, orange, cherry, crème, as well as colas. I'd grab a bottle, take the cap off with a bottle opener somewhere nearby and enjoy a refreshingly cold drink. Back then, the bottles held about six ounces of soda.

Nowadays, you go into a convenience store, grab a cup and fill it with a cold drink. But it's the size of the cup that is real difference. By modern standards, a 32-ounce drink is a small one. Typically, if you can get your arms all the way around the container it's still too small!

What's happened here? Are the people of today a lot more thirsty than they were 40 years ago? No, somehow the boundaries of common sense have been broken. We've come to believe that unless we get the biggest drink, the largest meal, or the greatest quantity for our money then we've been cheated.

So in search of the biggest bang for our dollar we order the huge drink, we hit the buffet line, or at a restaurant we get the appetizer, the meal *and* the dessert. Oh, we get our money's worth, all right. Far more than we need, and the consequences show up on our bathroom scales if we're brave enough to stand on them.

Our food portions have become a victim of ignoring boundaries. The CAMP system can restore those boundaries and give you real strategies for planning how you're going to eat a meal.

Finding Your Bite Size

How much food should you put in your mouth at one time? If you're trying to set a world's record you might attempt a dozen hot dogs at once. But if you're trying to bring some sanity to your eating you may want to take a close look at "bite size."

Bite size refers to the amount of food that you place in your mouth. Most of us rarely give this any thought. We just put food in our mouths, chew and swallow. End of story.

In the CAMP system, the ideal bite size is defined as *the smallest amount of food that makes sense.*

You could eat a cookie crumb by crumb, but chewing on a tiny crumb doesn't make much sense. You probably couldn't even taste it!

On the other hand, stuffing three cookies in your mouth at once isn't the right answer either. Other than overloading your mouth, you'd be ignoring Principle #10 that states that *Being in harmony and balance with food is part of living a life of dignity and grace.* It's difficult to imagine any dignity or grace in having three cookies jammed in one's mouth.

No, the perfectly sized bite is somewhere in between. Any smaller than perfect size and the bite's too small to chew. Any bigger than perfect size and you've taken more than you need to enjoy the food and the process of chewing it.

Here's another definition of the ideal bite size: *if you can chew the entire bite without feeling the need to swallow part of it, the bite size is correct.*

For many, the right bite size is really pretty small. This is a bonus of the CAMP system. You'll be taking smaller bites, your food will last much longer, and you'll be eating for a longer period. It also means that a *smaller amount of food* will seem like more, because you'll be eating it over a longer time.

The exercise below will help you find the right bite size for you.

Practice: Finding Your Bite Size

This practice will help you find how big a bite is the right amount of food for you. Along the way, you'll also have more practice in eating mindfully.

You will need one apple, a plate, a bottle or glass of water for clearing and a sharp knife. Find a time when you can devote 10 minutes or so to eating this apple.

Do not cut the apple up yet. Place the apple on the plate. Put the water next to it and have the knife nearby.

1.   First, let's arrive at this apple. Take a moment to really look at it. Notice its colors, its patterns and its shape. Understand that an apple is the swollen base of the apple flower (the receptacle of the flower).
2.   Notice its shine. The skin is a waterproof covering that preserves the apple. Feel its smoothness.

3. Does your apple have any odor?

4. Feel its weight in your hand. Much of that is due to the moisture content of the apple.

5. Find the old flower parts at the very bottom of the apple. The dried, wizened brown things there are the old petals.

6. Consider the apple stem at the top, which was the lifeline of the apple to the rest of the tree.

7. Think about this apple as an energy gift from the tree. Consider the many weeks it took to grow this apple and the effort of the tree to produce it.

8. Now, cut your apple into 20 or so pieces. The best way is to cut the apple in half through the stem. Then, cut each half in half, again top down. With each quarter, cut the core and seeds out and then cut from the center out to the skin many times, creating small pieces of apple each with some skin on it. During the first few bites you take, you're going to determine what is the appropriate bite size for you. If the first bite you take is too big, reduce it for the second bite. If a bite's too small, make the next one bigger. Get a sense of what bite size is right for you.

9. Now, eat a piece of the apple. During this first bite, chew your apple and taste the sweetness. Taste the sugars in your apple and realize that the sugar is stored energy from the sun. Chew your apple completely. Are you ready to swallow? Chew it three more times. Now swallow.

10. Clear with a small sip of water.

11. If the first bite was too big, make this bite smaller. Or make this bite a little bigger if the first bite was too small. Remember, you should be able to chew the whole bite completely before swallowing.

12. On this second bite, chew your apple and notice the tartness. This is the presence of a mild acid in the apple. As you chew, notice how the tartness changes. Are you ready to swallow? Chew three more times. Now swallow.

13. Clear.

14. Make any minor adjustments to your bite size on this bite. By now, you should be getting a pretty clear idea of what's right for you. Remember, the ideal size is small enough to still make sense. Make sure all the bites from now on are the same size (use the knife to cut pieces smaller if you have to).

15. Now chew the next bite and make sure your apple piece includes some of the skin. Separate out the taste of the skin from the taste of the flesh. How would you describe the taste of the skin? its density? its mouth feel? its chewability? Now swallow.

16. Clear.

17. The next bite will concentrate on the crunchiness of the apple. Notice its snap at first. How does it change as you chew? What sound does your apple make as you chew it? And how do these sounds change? Are you ready to swallow? Go ahead.

18. Clear.

19. This bite, pay attention to the texture of the apple. Before you chew, notice the edges of the apple your knife created. Are they completely smooth? A little rough? What about the feel of the apple skin on your tongue? Now chew, and follow the changes in texture. Swallow and clear.

20. This bite, pay attention to the juices you release as your chew. Can you feel the flow? Chew tight; make your teeth small cider presses. Extract all the flavorful juices. Flood you mouth with them. Swallow and clear.

21. How many chews does it take to chew up your bite of apple? Let's find out. With this apple bite, count the number of chews until the apple is completely chewed up. Swallow and clear.

22. With this bite, let's experiment with controlling our chew rate. Concentrate on chewing this bite of the apple at one half the normal speed. Count the number of times you chew. Be aware of every slow movement of your jaws. Don't rush; in fact, slow your chewing down as much as you can. When you're ready, swallow and then clear. What did you learn about how many chews are needed when you chew more slowly?

23. Now, let's go a little farther afield. With this bite, go deeper and taste the sun that shone on this apple, that gave up its energy, that ripened the apple. Can you taste the sun's force in the apple. Taste the sun…be poetic! Swallow and clear.

24. Go deeper. As you chew your apple, taste its journey from the orchard to you. Consider the basket that held it, the truck that moved it, the hand that stacked it. Follow its path in your mind with each chewing motion. Swallow and clear.

25. For the next bites as your finish your apple, explore and be creative. What does this apple mean to you? What does its taste evoke? What memories or associations does it stir? Enjoy this apple in silence, clearing after each bite. Relax….slow down….be attentive…take your time…be deliberate…have fun…feel in control….experience every bite….be in harmony….treat yourself well….be gracious….eat in dignity.

Learning your bite size will be a long-term experimentation, especially as you have experience with different foods. A bite of spaghetti may be slightly different that a bite of carrot or ice cream. Foods with more sugar or fat in them may require smaller bites. As you tune in to your body, you will learn what's right for you with all the foods.

Beverages Too

Beverages don't have bite sizes, but the same idea can be applied. Think of sips as controlling the amount of beverage you take in at one time. The right-sized sip is the smallest amount of liquid that makes sense. Too much fluid is simply gulping. Too little fluid is silly: drinking a soda drop by drop doesn't honor either the food portion of the soda or yourself.

Practice: The Cookie and Tea Encounter

This Tea and Cookie Practice gives you an opportunity to eat with the right bite sizes and drink with the right sip sizes.

During this encounter you will need one small cookie, a freshly brewed cup of tea and a glass or bottle of water for clearing. If you are accustomed to drinking coffee instead of tea, I would encourage you to drink tea anyway. The CAMP system urges you to try all foods and rediscover them. Remember: not everything we eat or drink has to be delicious. Simple foods can be appreciated for their gifts of sustenance beyond the flavors they possess.

Find a place to eat the cookie and drink the tea that has few distractions. Also, find a place where you can see a clock (or just use a wristwatch).

1. Fix yourself a cup of tea. Prepare it mindfully. Think about your actions as you boil the water, steep the tea and wait for it to brew. Let your mind settle solely on the act of making tea as much as possible.
2. You may add cream, sugar and lemon to your tea, but you may want to try just plain tea. Remember, not all foods have to taste sweet or creamy or have sharp flavors. Sometimes, simple is better.
3. Select a single small cookie and take it and your tea and water to where you're going to enjoy them.
4. Sit down and place the items in front of you. Arrive at your small snack. Take a moment and just relax. No hurry here. Think about the gifts of the tea and cookie, the efforts to produce them, the resources needed to grow the living things responsible. Notice the time on the clock; you're going to eat your single cookie and drink your tea over the next 10 minutes.
5. Begin to eat your cookie. First, smell it. Then, take a very small bite. Chew it extra slowly and carefully. Set the rest of the cookie down. Allow your mind to see the wheat fields from which the flour came to make this cookie. See the sugar cane that was the source of the cookie's sugar. Taste all aspects of your cookie. Notice its crunch, its chewability, its mix of flavors. Swallow carefully and feel the cookie enter your system.
6. Clear with a small sip of water.
7. After your first bite of cookie, sit quietly. No need to get to the tea in a hurry. Take pleasure in the experience. Dwell in the present. Make this act of enjoying your cookie and this tea last at least 10 minutes.

8. Now, take the teacup or mug in your hand. Feel its warmth. Bring the tea near your face. Feel the warmth and moisture rising. Smell the tea. Take a moment and just enjoy being near the tea.

9. Take a sip of tea. Just a sip. Let it stay in your mouth for a little while. Taste it, sense its warmth. Allow your mind to see the ocean, the vast source of water on our planet. See rain or snow or sleet, all the ways that water comes to us. Imagine a billion living things giving off water in the course of their lives. Be creative as you taste this tea. Let the tea linger on your tongue for a moment. Swallow and feel the tea go down your esophagus and enter your stomach. Experience the aftertastes of the tea. Slow down. Enjoy. Sit quietly and reflect on the tea.

10. Clear with water.

11. Continue eating your cookie and sipping your tea in this manner for at least 10 minutes, clearing after each bite or sip of tea. Place your full attention on the cookie and the tea. Keep your bites and sips very small. If you're a little bored or find yourself distracted, just bring your attention back to the tea and cookie. Resist turning on the TV or grabbing a magazine. Don't get unfocused or sidetracked. Make the eating of the cookie and the drinking of the tea a sacred act of dignity and honor.

12. When you are finished, pause and reflect on the experience. As you clean up, do so mindfully. Wash your teacup by hand, paying attention to the washing. Remind yourself that with the camp system, the entire process of eating, from preparation to clean up, can be a time of deliberateness and balance.

13. Add the tea and cookie to your Journal for today. Write about what you've learned. What was difficult about this exercise? What was enjoyable? What did you learn about how you were eating and drinking before?

Cutting Up Food

Once you find your bite size, you'll know what you can handle with each bite comfortably. You can translate that knowledge into action: from now on, you will cut up your food into bite-sized pieces.

Yes, it's true: we cut up food for youngsters and we may cut up food for the very old. But now we're going to cut up the food for ourselves. When we do, we help ourselves eat in a new way. We're going to pay attention to a small amount of food, bite by bite.

Cutting the food up at the beginning of a meal also helps us arrive at the meal. Before we begin eating, we have another job to do. We cut up the food carefully, mindfully, aware of the size of each bite we intend to eat.

We cut up the steak, the meatloaf, the baked potato. We cut up our green beans when they're too long or big for a single bite. We cut up our spaghetti or lasagna into bite-sized pieces.

We cut up our carrots, our fried chicken, our pizza. We know our bite size and we make sure that the food we eat is ready to go in the size we need.

We cut up our liver, our ham, our turkey, our fish. We cut up the pie, the cake, the apple dumpling. In short, we cut up anything that we can that makes sense to cut up into our bite size.

Loaves and Fishes

When we cut up our food, something amazing happens. You may have noticed when you cut up the apple to find your bite size that one apple suddenly became a plateful of food. This is an experience I respectfully call the "Loaves and Fishes Phenomenon." A small amount of food seems to change—almost miraculously—into a large amount. Half an apple, cut up, suddenly appears to be an entire lunch. Each piece of apple is its own bite. It will be eaten mindfully, slowly, deliberately. You look at the plate and realize that a small amount of food will take you 15 or 20 minutes to eat. Your brain smiles, knowing that it will be experiencing the pleasure of eating for a long time (even though the amount of food is relatively small).

I've also found that something else takes place when I cut up food into bite-sized pieces. After a while, I actually get tired of eating. Forty minutes of sitting at dinner, eating and clearing, is a long time, and often I don't finish my plate simply because I'm growing weary of eating that particular meal.

Cutting up your food will automatically begin to limit the amount you're eating. Each bite on the plate will remind you to slow down and eat mindfully. And there's no need to hold on to your silverware during the meal, because the food's already cut up.

Exceptions

Of course not all foods can be cut up. Creamed corn, ice cream, tapioca and pudding all demand to be eaten one spoonful at a time. But you're in control—you decide how much goes on the spoon and how long you enjoy the food in your mouth before you swallow.

On the Go

Eating on the run presents its own problems. What do you do when the only choice is a burger and fries at the local fast food place and you're going to eat while on the road? Sandwiches are usually not cut up to eat. And the fries come to you in the little cardboard box ready to be plucked out with the fingers.

If you can't cut up your food, remember your bite size anyway. Take small bites of your sandwich that still make sense. See how long you can make the sandwich last. If you really like burgers and fries, this is a great way to extend your enjoyment. Take the fries one at a time. If the fry is too long, bite it in half and just chew that part (putting the other half back for later). Don't let the inability to cut up the food stop you from eating in the CAMP way!

Practice: Cutting up Food

Starting with your next meal, cut up any foods that can be cut up. Don't begin eating until the foods are cut into bite sizes. Cut the food carefully, being aware of your muscles moving and the process of how you decide how small the pieces will be.

Notice how the food expanded on your plate. Consider that each piece of food is a separate bite, requiring you to be attentive, mindful and careful. As you eat, take one morsel of food at a time. Put your silverware down and bring your attention to each bite (for a second, at least) as you chew.

Don't forget to clear with water after each and every bite.

Commit to reaching for your knife at the beginning of each meal. Make the act of cutting the food part of your arrival at the meal.

You know how I feel about pizza, and this book wouldn't be complete without a practice involving that wonderful food. This next practice uses pizza to give you more experience with cutting up food.

Practice: Pizza

Pizza is the universal food in many situations, and sooner or later pizza will probably come into your life. Rather than avoid it and turn to some boring, low-fat salad, why not enjoy your pizza in the CAMP way?

This Practice assumes that you have at least several pieces of a good, thick-crusty pizza, but any type of pizza will do. Don't forget your beverage and water for clearing

1. Arrive at the pizza. The standard pizza is a gift of wheat, tomatoes, cheese (thank the cow) and smaller amounts of other ingredients. If you have toppings on your pizza, there are even more gifts to consider. Reflect on all the efforts to get pizza to your table. Think about how you're going to eat your pizza.

2. Put a single piece of pizza on your plate. Cut up the non-crust portion of your pizza into bite sizes. If you have a slab of crust remaining, leave it for later.

3. Take a small bite of pizza each time, slowly chewing and enjoying it. Savor the full flavors, aromas and textures of your pizza. If you have toppings, pay attention to the separate flavors, textures and blends. Swallow only when the bite of pizza is fully chewed.

4. After each bite, clear with water.

5. After each drink of beverage, clear with water.

6. Pause between bites and extend the pleasurable experience of eating pizza as long as you like.

7. If you have a crust uneaten, cut up the crust into bite-sized pieces. The crust may not be as flavorful as the other portion of the slice, but still it has gifts of energy and nutrition. Eat the crust slowly, deliberately, mindfully, a bite at a time. Force yourself to appreciate the food. Clear between bites.

8. Consider the end of the first slice as a boundary, a stopping point to ask yourself where your HQ is and how much more you may want. If your body needs more food, by all means get more pizza. Eat the second slice in the same way as you did the first. No need to rush. Stay in the present moment and accept all the gifts the pizza offers.

9. At the end of the second slice, you've reached another boundary. Ask yourself if you need more. Then, ask yourself if you really need more. Trust that your body will tell you the truth. If you need another piece of pizza, go for it.

Portion Strategies

There are four basic portions strategies that are part of the CAMP system. They are:

- The Two Plate strategy
- The Double Circle strategy
- The Counter strategy
- The Buddy strategy

All of these methods help you set boundaries for yourself and can be used just about anywhere.

The Two Plate Strategy

This is my favorite strategy and I use it frequently, especially in restaurants, where I don't have control over how much food is on the plate to begin with. I also use this method with salads, especially when they are served in bowls or on plates that are far too small for eating the salad comfortably.

This method creates boundaries by using two plates instead of one. The space between the two plates is a large, visible, unavoidable boundary you want to approach with great care.

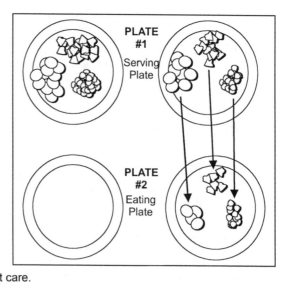

1. Start with a plate of food. Before you cut the food up, set your plate back away from you on the table and get another plate. This second plate can be the same size as the first plate, but it's even better if it's a smaller plate. Your original plate (the one with all the food on it) is now your Serving Plate, and the new plate is your Eating Plate.

2. From your serving plate, take some of each food and place it on your camp Plate. Just how much to take you'll have to decide, but trust yourself to put a portion on the plate that makes sense.

3. Cut up the food on your Eating Plate into bite-sized pieces.

4. Eat all the food on your Eating Plate—slowly, mindfully, thoughtfully, eating it in the CAMP way and clearing after each bite.

5. When you're done with all the food on the Eating plate, stop. Evaluate. Ask yourself: Do I need more? Do I really need more? If not, you're done. If you do need more, go on to the next step.

6. Bring half the food from the Serving Plate onto your Eating Plate. Cut this food up and eat it.

7. Again, stop and evaluate. The idea here is to make deliberate decisions at stopping points during the meal, frequently evaluating if you need more food. How often will you cross the boundary between the two plates? How much food is really enough?

8. If you need more food, repeat steps 6 and 7.

Try the Two Plate strategy at buffets. Put food on one plate and carry an extra plate back to the table with you. You'll be amazed how long the food lasts from your first trip to the buffet. You just may not have to go back for that second plate.

Without any hesitation, I routinely ask for extra plates at restaurants. I've never been treated rudely for this; usually, my waitperson is glad to bring extra plates.

Mentioned in the Two Plate strategy was the idea of stopping at several points in the meal to see if you "really need more." What does this mean? How does one evaluate if one needs more food?

Knowing When to Quit

The answer is in tuning to your HQ (hunger quotient). You learned about your HQ in chapter 9, where you rated your hunger on a ten-point scale (1 for famished, 10 for not hungry at all).

It is here in the Portions part of CAMP that the HQ becomes important. When you stop eating in the middle of a meal to see if you need more food, you need to look at your HQ. If you've had enough food just where should your HQ be?

If you keep eating until your HQ is at a 9 or 10, you've gone too far. (In all the months and months I've been on the CAMP system, I've never eaten to the point where I felt "stuffed.") At the end of a meal, you should be able to leave the table feeling fine, energetic and comfortable.

You might even decide to leave the table while still feeling a little hungry. Here's how it works: During a meal, some of the food you ate at the beginning has already digested in your system. But the food you ate most recently is still in your stomach. It's going to take another 10, 20 or 30 minutes for it to get digested and distributed by your blood. If you leave the table a little hungry, it's likely that a half an hour later you'll feel fine. That's because by then all your food will have entered your system.

What's right for you? Only you can say. And the only way you can find out is to experiment. Force yourself to end a meal a little early with your HQ at a 4 or 5. Then, notice in 20 minutes or so: has your HQ gone up? Are you still hungry? (If so, get more food!)

Ideally, when you're in balance with food you'll be able to keep your HQ between 3 and 7 all the time. Before meals, you'll feel slightly hungry but rarely famished. After meals, you'll feel comfortable or a little full but never stuffed.

The Rule of 20

The idea of waiting 20 minutes when hungry is a handy rule and can give you a sense of control over your hunger. In the 20 minutes after a meal, changes are still occurring in your body. By waiting that extra time, you may find you don't need that second helping or the dessert you thought you did.

But the Rule of 20 can be applied in other situations as well. I tell my CAMP students: "Anytime you feel hungry and are tempted to get a snack, wait 20 minutes. If you still feel hungry, go ahead and get your snack, but be sure to eat in the CAMP way." I know from experience that when you feel hungry, that hunger triggers the mind to ask for food. When it doesn't get food in the stomach (because you're waiting 20 minutes), the brain turns elsewhere for energy, usually to stored fat. So by waiting 20 minutes, you instruct the brain to burn off the stored energy you've wanted to lose anyway. The brain is happy (it's found food) and you're happy (you're losing weight and you don't feel hungry anymore).

So: Anytime you feel hungry and are tempted to get a snack, wait 20 minutes. If you still feel hungry, go ahead and get your snack, but be sure to eat in the CAMP way.

The Double Circle Strategy

This strategy works well when you can't easily get extra plates.

This strategy allows you to create boundaries as you divide your food on the plate. At first, the boundaries will be visible on the plate, but later on you'll know where the boundaries are even it you don't separate your food.

1. Before you begin a meal, cut up your food. Let's say you're going to eat a meal of meatloaf, mashed potatoes and green beans. Cut up your meatloaf into bite-sized pieces. Also, cut up any large green beans to make them bite sized as well. (It really doesn't make sense to cut up the mashed potatoes!) Now consider each type of food on your plate. Take your knife and draw a line halfway down the cut-up meatloaf. Move one-half towards the center of the plate and push the remaining amount towards the edge. Do the same for the potatoes and the beans. When you're done, you should have a cluster of

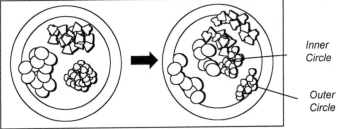

Inner
Circle

Outer
Circle

food in the center of the plate and piles of food at the edge. The space between the pile is the physical boundary you've created.

2. Eat from the outer circle at the edges of the plate. Eat all the food in the CAMP way—slowly, mindfully, thoughtfully. Clear after each bite.

3. Finish all the food from the outer circle. When you're done, stop. Evaluate. Ask yourself: Do I need more? Where is my HQ? Do I really need more? If not, you're done. Don't be afraid to throw the rest away or keep it as leftovers. If you do need more, go on to the next step.

4. Take your knife and draw a line through each of the piles at the center of the plate. Move one half of each pile to the edge. You're dividing your food again, making new physical boundaries.

5. Now eat this food from the outer edge of the plate, mindfully, slowly, deliberately. When you're done with all food in the center, stop. Evaluate. Ask yourself: Do I need more? Do I really need more? If not, you're done. If you do need more, go on to the next step. (You may at this point decide to wait 20 minutes before going on.)

6. Continue dividing your food, bringing more from the center and eating from the outer circle. The idea is to continue to set up visible boundaries and to give yourself an idea of how much food you really need.

7. If you've eaten all the food on your plate and you still really need more, get more, but follow the same procedure of creating boundaries in the food.

8. After using this method for some time, you'll be able to see the boundaries without physically dividing the food. You'll know what your portions should be, and you'll be on your way to finding your own harmony and balance.

The Counter Strategy

With this method, the source of the food stays elsewhere—on a counter or on the stove-top perhaps, but not on the dinner table. The boundaries you create are very large, possibly a full room away or even farther.

1. All the food stays in the kitchen, either on the stove or on a counter. Don't put any food on the table where you're going to eat. Leave the butter, salt, jelly, etc. away from the table.

2. Put a small amount of food on your plate there and move to the table (or another location) to eat it. It's important that you select intentionally small portions to begin with here.

3. Eat the food on your plate in the CAMP way. Don't forget to clear after each bite. When you are finished, ask yourself if you need more. Evaluate your HQ. Then ask yourself if you really need more. If not, you're done. If so, move on to the next step.

4. Return to the counter to get more food. This is a deliberate act that required walking and carrying your plate. Each decision to get up and get more food means crossing the boundary.

5. Again take a small amount of food.

6. Return to the place where you're eating and finish this next serving. When you are finished, ask yourself if you need more. If so, you're done, but if not, you may want to continue. (You may at this point decide to wait 20 minutes before continuing to eat.)

7. Continue on this way until your body tells you that you've had enough.

CAMP Buddy strategy

A CAMP buddy is someone else who is also using the CAMP system. It may be a friend, a co-worker, a spouse, or life partner. By teaming with your buddy, you both create boundaries defined by each other's plate.

- **At a restaurant**, order a single meal and share it. Ask for extra plates—most restaurants are eager to comply. Eat your food in the CAMP way. Then, when you're done, evaluate. Do you need more food? Do you *really* need more? If not, you're done. But if you think you'd like more, then by all means order more (or, even better, wait 20 minutes before ordering more). Perhaps get a dessert (many restaurants feed you so much you may rarely have room for dessert; now you can try some!). Better still—split the dessert with your buddy. Again, when you're done evaluate. Still need more? Then order another dessert. My guess is, though, that you won't need more.

- **At home**, prepare a single meal and split it. If you eat frozen dinners from time to time, just heat one and split it. Then, when you're done, evaluate. Do you need more food? Do you *really* need more? If not, you're done. But if you think you'd like more, then prepare more food. Often, one meal will be enough for you *and* your buddy.

The Buddy Strategy is wonderful because you get support from another CAMPer, someone with whom you can share not only your food but your struggles, ideas, concerns and successes as well.

One of the most important lessons I've learned from experimenting with portions is that the amount of food I *really* needed each day wasn't very much at all. The truth is that *all we need for each meal is enough food to get us to the next meal.* What you eat for breakfast should get you to lunch. What you eat for lunch should get you to dinner. What you eat for dinner should get you to breakfast the next morning. All the rest is unnecessary. By creating boundaries in your eating, you can learn what is right for you.

Progress

At this point in the CAMP system you are:

❑ Continuing your daily food Journal.
❑ Continuing to evaluate to whom or to what you're giving up power over food and seeing yourself daily on the Food Economy diagram.
❑ Reviewing the ten CAMP Principles every day.
❑ Arriving at food of every meal.
❑ Eating with mindfulness, care, attentiveness, if only for a second each bite.
❑ Putting your silverware (or any food in your hand) down as you chew.
❑ Tuning in to your body, its needs, its enjoyment, it motions and its feelings.
❑ Bringing mindfulness to getting food, preparing food, setting the table, cleaning up, putting dishes away, etc.
❑ Challenging just about everything to do with how you were eating in the past by becoming aware of how you eat, how fast, how long you pause between bites, etc.
❑ Clearing after every bite with a sip of water.
❑ Using one or more of the Portions strategies, creating visible boundaries in your food. You're evaluating how much you eat at each boundary.

14.

The Complete CAMP System

As the last chapter drew to a close, you received the last steps of the complete CAMP system. You now have all the information to be a total CAMPer, each and every meal of the day for all of your days. It may now be several weeks or more since you started with chapter 1. If you've done all the practice exercises and kept up with your Journal, you've already developed many skills and insights. Ideally, your sense of control of food is becoming stronger and stronger, and you're finding yourself much more in harmony and balance with food than ever before.

The purpose of this chapter is to summarize the steps of the CAMP system. As part of that, I've included four new practice exercises to help you in most circumstances.

The first practice is a general sequence of steps you could use with most any meal. If you need a refresher from time to time, this practice may be the best place to start.

The three other practices in this chapter give you suggestions for other eating situations: eating a salad, going to a buffet and dropping in at your local fast-food restaurant.

First, though, here's a very basic summary of the CAMP system:

The CAMP System

1. Arrive at the food. Notice its colors, shapes, aromas. Consider its gifts. Imagine eating the food. Be thankful.

2. Cut the food up into bite-sized pieces. Foods you can't cut you will eat with small bites.

3. Create boundaries in the food. Select food to eat first and leave the rest for later servings.

4. Eat each bite mindfully. Chew the food completely. For at least one second during each bite, turn your spotlight on the food.

5. During each bite, put your silverware down. Don't hold any food in your hands while chewing.

6. Once you've chewed the food completely, swallow slowly.

7. After each bite, clear the palate with water. Treat all other beverages as food.

8. Pause after each clearing. Enjoy your meal.

9. At some point, pause and evaluate how you feel. Do you need more food? If so, take more. If not, stop eating.

10. If possible, stop eating while you're still a little hungry. Your hunger should go away after you digest more of your food.

11. Whenever you have hunger pangs, let them go for 20 minutes. If they still nag at you after that time, get some food. Remember: *feeling a little hunger (emptiness) means that the system is working and that your body is burning stored food.*

12. Extend your mindfulness to any activity having to do with food.

13. Use this procedure any time you eat—meals, snacks, treats, anything.

14. Write in your CAMP Journal every day.

Practice: The Basic CAMP Meal

This sequence of steps could be used for most meals. The most important thing to remember here is that the CAMP system is all about control. You are in control. You will decide how much, how fast and how long you will eat. You will decide how long to wait between bites, how slowly you will chew or how many times you will chew. Virtually everything about food and eating is in your power to control.

1. Gather the food for your meal mindfully, whether you're just taking a box out of a cabinet, shopping for food or hunting for your meal. All are equally important.

2. Set the table with deliberateness and care.

3. Prepare the meal with the sense of the sacred. Give honor to the food at every step. No matter if you're pouring cereal from a carton or creating a full Thanksgiving dinner from scratch—the tasks are equally worthy.

4. Be sure to include water at the meal for clearing.

5. Just before you begin to eat, stop. Pause. Arrive. Consider the food, its colors and aromas, its shapes and histories. Imagine yourself eating the food and the strategies you'll use.

6. Cut up all the food that can be cut up. Make the pieces bite sized.

7. Create boundaries in your food. Use two plates or divide the food on your plate. Share your food with a friend or leave the food on the counter and put some on your plate. Decide now where you'll stop to evaluate if you need more food.

8. As you begin eating, eat one bite at a time. As you start to chew, empty your hands.

9. Chew thoroughly, slowly, on purpose. Wake up! Bring the spotlight of your consciousness to the food. Be aware of the taste, texture, odors and the feel of food in your mouth. Think about where the food came from and its gift of energy. Consider the effort to get the food to your plate and all the people that contributed. For at least one second during each bite, eat mindfully.

10. Swallow slowly and attentively. Notice the aftertastes. Enjoy your food.

11. After each bite, clear with a small sip of water. Clean your palate and get it ready for the next bite.

12. Treat all beverages as food, and clear after each drink.

13. Pause between bites. There's no hurry now. Food is too precious and too valuable to rush. Your pause after each bite is a time to reflect on the present moment and the great gift before you.

14. When you reach the boundary you've created, stop and evaluate. Tune in to your body and trust what it tells you. If you need more food, by all means

have more. Continue by creating new boundaries and enjoying more food. If you don't need more, it's time to stop eating.

15. When you are finished, clear the table with concentration and purposefulness. Wash and dry the dishes mindfully, attentively. Put the dishes away as if they were prized relics from antiquity. Handle all the tools of eating with your greatest respect.

For most of your meals the procedure above should work well, whether you're eating at home or out at a restaurant. Some of the items may not exactly apply, but the essential elements to eating in the CAMP way are all there.

Salads

If you've ever been on a diet, you probably went through a salad stage. This is a state of mind where you think that just by eating lots of salad you'll reach some weight-reduction goal. It can work, but the strategy is full of land mines. Three of the worst of these are:

1. Over time you add "interesting" foods to the salads, such as meat, cheese, and eggs. The theory here (I guess) is that by mixing them with the lettuce and carrots, they somehow magically become less caloric, less fatty and less dangerous! Is it possible that lettuce turns the cheese calories into lettuce calories, making it all safe?

2. You choose sensible low-calorie veggies for the salad and then obliterate it all with hefty portions of salad dressing so that each piece is swimming in its own private pond of dressing. Or, you use a low-fat dressing but, figuring it's low in fat, you use twice as much, thereby bringing the fat content right back up.

3. You eat huge, mammoth, bowl-overflowing salads. This was my favorite strategy for a long time. I thought that if I filled up on salads, I'd eat less of the "regular" food. What I didn't realize at the time was that I was teaching myself to eat huge quantities of food during a meal, much, much more that I ever needed.

The next Practice will give you a new look at salads. When we apply the full CAMP system to eating a salad, we give ourselves wonderful, life-long opportunities to investigate foods in ways we haven't before.

Practice: A CAMP Salad

Salads are a wonderful way to get fresh vegetables. Although salads are quite popular, there are legions of people who don't like them. With the CAMP system, however, salads are worth another look.

Salads give you much to explore with mindful eating. Consider that salads are a generous mix of many foods. Each bite of a salad contains different tastes, textures, colors, aromas, and crunch factors. Every forkful can be a grand medley and a treasure trove of taste experiences. Begin to see the salad as new country to explore through mindfulness.

For this exercise, you will need a salad. Mindfully fix yourself a high-quality salad, full of good and diverse ingredients. A good way to do this is to visit a supermarket with a good salad bar. Start with tasty lettuce—let's face it: iceberg lettuce is not much more interesting than crunchy water. Try other types of lettuce, along with raw spinach. Beyond that, add tomatoes, cucumbers, peppers, celery, radishes, onions, chickpeas, baby corn, carrots, olives, snow peas, beets and pickles for starters. You may have other foods you prefer; go ahead and add them (but for now leave out the meats, cheeses and eggs). Throw in some croutons or sunflower seeds. Be creative and have fun.

The dressing you add to your salad can make or break the experience. I used to use low-fat or no-fat dressings on my salads and, in my opinion, nothing could be a bigger salad turnoff. Here's what I do now: I use regular salad dressing, but add only enough to coat everything. It's not necessary to float your salad in dressing!

Add a little of your favorite dressing (the kind you crave), mindfully stir it in, and cut up your salad, working the dressing in well until everything has a thin but noticeable covering on it. Bring your salad and water (for clearing) to where you're going to eat it.

Now you're ready for the CAMP Salad.

1. Fully arrive at your salad. Notice all the colors and textures. Think about all the efforts to get that salad to your bowl.
2. Mindfully find one item at a time with your fork and taste each item singly. Put just some lettuce in your mouth and experience it. Put your fork down.

3. Chew the lettuce thoroughly and slowly. Notice the taste and texture. Swallow, and notice the aftertastes. Pause and enjoy your eating experience. Then clear.

4. Next, find a tomato slice and eat it in the same way as above.

5. Next, find another type of food in your salad. The idea here is to experience each food by itself. Be sure to eat slowly and deliberately. Clear between bites. Continue on this way until you have sampled a bite of each and every type of food in your salad.

6. Now, try salad foods in combinations. Choose two types of food, say, a carrot slice and a cucumber slice, and put both on your fork and then into your mouth. Chew them together, but try to separate the tastes in your mouth. Can you taste the carrot? Can you taste the cucumber? Can you experience the texture of each? The crunch of each? Now notice how the tastes blend together. Do they create a third taste unique to the combination? Chew slowly and purposely. Swallow carefully and notice aftertastes. And, of course, clear after each bite.

7. After this first combination, try another and another and another. You may want to combine the carrot with all the other foods, or try new food combinations each time. With all the food types in your salad, you can sample different combinations for many, many bites. Keep your mind on your food, tasting carefully and honoring the food with your attention. Clear after each bite. Pause after each bite and reflect on the food.

8. If you like, try three types of food on your fork. Can you separate them in your mouth? Can you taste new combinations? The combinations and permutations are virtually endless.

9. Try this: before you put any food on your fork, close your eyes. Then, without looking, put food on your fork. Bring the food to your nose. Can you tell by odor what food is on your fork? Put the food in your mouth without opening your eyes. Can you tell what foods you are chewing? Chew slowly and carefully. Enjoy your salad. Repeat this process a number of times, clearing after each bite. Explore your salad as you would a new island.

10. When you have had enough salad (you don't have to eat it all!), push the bowl away from you in an act that signals you are done.

11. Reflect on your salad and the many gifts it has given you: energy, nutrition, protection from disease, fiber, enjoyment.

12. Clean up mindfully, handling carefully the tools of your eating.

The Real CAMP Challenge

When I teach the CAMP course, I use one class period to take my students out to a restaurant for a meal together. But I don't pick just any restaurant. I find the biggest, most appealing buffet I can find.

Why? Because buffets are one of the toughest places to eat. The food is plentiful and cheap, the choices are extensive, and usually the food is excellent.

I consider buffets to be temples of self indulgence. All boundaries are invisible. You can have as much as you want for as long as you want. No one is there to say "no." We're all kids in a candy store with no parent in sight.

Buffets work like this: we pay our money and then, for the next hour, we do everything we can to "get our money's worth." We begin at the salad bar, assembling a salad that two lumberjacks would have difficulty eating. And that's just for starters.

Next come the main courses: ham, steak, prime rib, shrimp, and king crab legs. Add the potatoes, pasta, bread and (if there's room) maybe some vegetables. We wolf all of this down as fast as possible to get in line again because—who knows—they might run out of crab legs!

After seconds and thirds, it's off to the dessert table and the ice cream machine, where we build ourselves a tower of delight. Then, back to the table to eat it all. We loosen our belts and think to ourselves: yes, we got our $9.99 worth out of that one, but if we can arrive at the buffet a little hungrier and a little emptier the next time we probably could eat even more.

There *is* a better way. The CAMP system will give you a new view of the buffet. Fully in control, you won't ever again have to feel in the irresistible grip of the buffet line. The next practice will give you a step-by-step approach to deal with buffets, pot lucks, parties, family reunions—anywhere with an abundance of food choices and the task of helping yourself.

I urge you to take this book to a buffet restaurant and work through the steps. You will win, not the buffet.

Practice: At the Buffet

There are many buffet restaurants in this country, and most of them are packed from the time they open to the time they close. Their overwhelming popularity is based on the perception that they offer the best value for the money. As a CAMPer, however, you don't have to be pulled in to that thinking.

To successfully approach a buffet line requires a re-ordering of thinking. It's important that you make two agreements with yourself:

A. **There is no way you can eat everything here today.** CAMP principle #4 states that there will always be more food. There will be other days, other meals, when you can return and try other foods. Agree with yourself that you're going to happy to sample only a small part of what you see.

B. **You're not going to get your money's worth with this meal.** Food is actually so cheap that you could never get the value commensurate with what you paid. Agree to think of the money you've paid for this buffet as your admission fee—it let you in the door, nothing more.

Now, on to the buffet:

1. **Beverage**: When you're seated in the restaurant, the server may ask you for your beverage choice. Order your beverage, and make sure to include water (for clearing) in your order.

2. **Arriving**: Head for the buffet, but before you fully get there, stop. Take it all in. Completely arrive at the buffet. See all the choices. Walk up and down the buffet tables slowly and examine all the foods there. Think about all the plants and animals that contributed to this array of food. Consider the human effort to prepare and assemble all this food. Create in your heart a feeling of gratitude for the food and that you can be here to enjoy it. As you walk, decide what you're going to eat this time during your visit.

3. When you're ready, take a plate and begin serving yourself.

4. **Salad**: If you're going to start with a salad, place the food in your salad bowl. Take a small portion. Remember, you can always come back if you want more salad. Before you take your salad back to the table, grab another salad bowl—you'll eat this salad with the Two-plate Strategy (see **Eating** below).

5. **Meal**: If you're starting with the main meal, take a regular size plate and make your food selections. Choose small portions. You can always come back if your need more. You are in control. Before you take your plate back to the table, grab another plate (a smaller one if possible), because you'll eat your meal with the Two-plate Strategy.

6. **Eating**: Place your food (serving) plate away from you and place your eating plate in front of you. Bring part of your salad or meal from the far plate to the near plate. Cut up all foods that can be cut up. Eat the food slowly, mindfully,

gratefully, deliberately. Empty your hands between bites. Chew thoroughly. Clear after all bites and sips of beverage. Pause after clearing.

7. **Evaluation**: When you've finished the food on your eating plate, stop and ask yourself if you need more. If not, consider a little dessert (below). If so, take more food from your serving plate and put in on your eating plate. Continue eating.

8. **Seconds**: If you finish all the food on your eating plate and still need more, have seconds. (Before you go for seconds, think: buffets are designed to entice you to have more food than you need. The buffet will be here tomorrow. Tune in to your body and find out what it really needs.) When you take seconds, take even smaller servings than you did before. Continue the Two-plate Strategy at the table. Remember: it will not hurt you to leave the buffet slightly hungry! Twenty minutes from now you probably won't be hungry. Don't be compelled to eat until you feel your stomach stretch. By then, it's too late—you've eaten more than you need.

9. **Dessert** - When you're done with the main part of the meal, you may have room for dessert. If you select pie, cake, fruit, etc., take a plate with dessert on it and an empty plate. Follow the Two-plate strategy at the table. If you select ice cream, put one-half the normal amount of ice cream in your bowl (you're using the Counter Strategy). Finish the smaller portion of ice cream and only then go back for the second half if you really need it.

Buffets are great places to watch other people eat, and if you can do so without staring you might give it a try. You will see all kinds of interesting eating behaviors. But resist the temptation to become judgmental, and don't start feeling superior to all the non-CAMPers there. It's dangerous to make assumptions about what other people need in their lives or what their relationships to food should be. Each person has his or her own path to follow. And besides, you're too busy caring for yourself and developing your own CAMP way to worry about how other are eating. Still, when you see how others eat, you can see it as if you are looking into a kind of mirror. Many of the behaviors you see were yours not so long ago. You truly have come far, haven't you?

Fast Foods

From the very start I knew that I wanted to write something in this book about eating at a fast food restaurant. Millions of people visit these establishments every day, and yet to my knowledge there have never been any instructions written on how to eat there sensibly. And there's also a delicious irony to the idea that any book that discusses weight loss would include a section on eating at a fast food restaurant. The very idea!

The first CAMP principle states that we should never be deprived. Of *course* you should feel free to go to a fast food restaurant—the food there is for your enjoyment. But that food has *special* gifts of energy, and we want to approach it with care.

Fast foods have not received favorable press in recent years, with reports of the high fat and calorie content of hamburgers, fried chicken and French fries. And yet, CAMP principle #3 states that all food is special and merits our deepest respect. Fast food is no different; we can honor the great gifts that fast food has to offer just as we honor other foods. Because most of the foods at a fast food restaurant are rich in fats and carbohydrates, we want to take extra care and give extra honor to the abundant gifts they bring us.

The next time you visit a fast food restaurant, take this book with you and work through the next practice. You may want to try this alone so you can explore your own strategies for enjoying this common American experience.

Practice: Fast Food

This practice assumes that you are going to order a hamburger with all the fixin's (including cheese and bacon), a small order of fries (you can, you know, always order more fries if you need them), a regular soft drink and a dessert. If you order foods other than these, read along anyway and make your own modifications in the text for the foods of your choice.

You will also need a timepiece—a simple wristwatch will do. Finally, a sharp food knife may be helpful. You could carry a small, serrated food knife wrapped in a handkerchief to restaurants when the tools there are inadequate to cutting food.

1. Place your order. Don't forget to order both a beverage and water (for clearing). It's okay to just order water. Bring your food to the table and sit down.
2. Arrive at the food. Consider all the plants and animals who have made sacrifices for you to eat here today. Here's a partial list:

> Cow: its muscle ground up is hamburger, its milk forms cheese.
> Pig: its muscles and fat make up the bacon.
> Tomato: you're going to eat the fruit of the plant, also in the ketchup.
> Lettuce: you're going to eat the leaves of the plant.

Onion: you're going to eat the underground stem of the plant.
Cucumber: a pickle is the preserved fruit of the plant.
Potato: the fries are sliced underground stems.
Apple: it's in the vinegar in the ketchup.
Corn: its syrup is in the ketchup.
Wheat: its ground up dried fruits form flour, used to make the bun and
   the crust of the dessert pie.
Sesame: its seeds are toasted and are on the bun.
Peanut: its oil is heated and is used to fry the fries.

3. Cut your hamburger. Don't cut it up into little pieces; instead, cut it in half, but cut it a little off center. This will create a larger half and a smaller half. You're going to start with the large half and save the small half for later. During your arrival at the food, consider that it's possible that you'll throw the small half away. (CAMP principle #6 states that it's better to leave food uneaten than to eat more than is needed.)

4. Take your fries and on your tray divide them into two piles: a larger pile and a smaller pile. You're going to eat from the larger pile. Decide during your arrival at the food that you may throw away the small pile of fries.

5. Look at your watch or clock and note the time. Your task is to eat the larger half of your hamburger and the larger pile of fries in a way to make them last 20 minutes.

6. Take small bites of the hamburger. Chew each bite thoroughly. Take your time. Give honor to the food. Enjoy your food. Taste all the many tastes.

7. Clear after each bite.

8. Take small bites of your fries. Most fries are too big to eat in one bite. Experiment with your bite size and find the smallest bite that makes sense. Pick up a French fry, bite off your bite amount and put the rest of the fry down. Enjoy slowly and mindfully. Clear after each bite.

9. Take sips of your beverage. Don't gulp. Sip, enjoy, swallow. Clear after each sip.

10. Pause generously after each bite. Notice aftertastes. Don't hurry. Stretch out your experience here to last 20 minutes.

11. As the end of 20 minutes approaches, you may have to eat faster or slower, depending on how much of your food is left. At the 20-minute mark, stop. You've eaten the larger half of your hamburger, the larger pile of your French fries, and some of your beverage. Now is the time to evaluate: Do you need more? Do you really need more? Where is your HQ? Keep in mind that you have dessert ahead, so factor it into your decision. Ask yourself: What if there was an emergency right now and I had to leave quickly at this point? Would I have had enough food? Would I survive to the next meal? Just what makes sense?

12. If you stop eating your meal here, wrap up the remaining hamburger and fries. Throw them away. Go on to eat your dessert.

13. If you need more food, cut the remaining hamburger in half. Make two piles from the remaining fries. Look at your timepiece and force yourself to take five minutes to eat half of the hamburger and one small pile of fries. Really slow it down. Take even smaller bites. Chew slower. Intensify your mindfulness. Clear and pause after each bite.

14. At the end of five minutes, stop. Look at the food remaining. Be thankful for the experience, wrap up the hamburger and fries that are left and throw them away. You will never miss them.

15. Unwrap your dessert and arrive at it. Give yourself five minutes to eat this dessert. Clear after each bite. But after every bite, ask yourself if you need more. There is no law that says you have to finish this dessert. After the fourth bite, you should have your cravings satisfied. (Remember the Rule of Four?) Commit that you will throw at least one bite of the dessert away. If you're still eating at the end of five minutes, throw away any food or beverage left.

This Fast Food practice can be extremely empowering. You leave the restaurant feeling in control. You've made all the decisions about how to eat food that once may have had uncontested power over you. From this point on, you never have to feel in the powerless grip of fast foods again.

Your course has now been set. You know what to do for every meal, every snack, every encounter with food ahead.

No matter if you're eating a hot dog at the ballpark or you're facing a Thanksgiving dinner. No matter if you're at home or traveling. No matter if you're facing holiday cookies at the office or eating with friends at the buffet. You have all the skills and strategies to last you the rest of your life in any eating situation. You have gathered back your power over food, and you no longer give away control to anyone or anything else.

If you're watching your weight, you very well may be seeing changes. When you reach the weight you want to be—that your body tells you is right for you—there are still a few tasks ahead.

15.

Balance and Harmony (Maintenance)

The CAMP system came into being because I needed to lose weight. And lose weight I did. As I approached the weight where my body told me it should be, I had to shift my eating a little to bring it into a balanced state.

Think back to the Simple Food Economy diagram on page 37. During the time I was losing weight, I stayed in diagram C, taking in less energy than I was using. My body found the extra energy and burned it off.

But when I reached my goal, I had to move to diagram B. Day by day, I wanted the energy I took in to equal (more or less) the energy I was using. This is the equilibrium point, and one of many things that indicates a living in balance with food.

Balance...

Frankly, I was amazed at how much more food I had to eat to reach the balance point. The first week I thought I ate more and indeed my Journal showed me that I had increased my food intake. It wasn't enough; I still lost some weight.

The next week I added more food to my meals. Still not enough—a few more pounds had come off.

Only by experimentation, meal by meal, week by week, did I finally reach the amount that was right for me.

Since reaching my goal many month ago my weight has been steady. I weigh myself once a week, and if I see a slight increase or decrease I compensate slightly during the following week.

And just in case you think that I'm super careful just because I've written this book, you should know that I eat dinner out three or four times a week and I have lunches out usually twice a week. I eat the foods I love and never feel deprived. Being in balance with food is terrific!

...and Harmony

The other aspect of the CAMP system is being in harmony with food. During the last year and a half, while the CAMP system was being developed, I found myself changing significantly in my eating style and food preferences. I didn't realize it at the time, but now I know these shifts and changes were all a part of realigning my body, mind and spirit with food.

If my experience and the experience of my clients and students is typical, here are a few changes you might see in yourself over the next months:

- Your tastes in food will change. I find myself drawn to vegetables more and more, enjoying them to the fullest. Rarely do I go to fast food restaurants anymore, not because anyone told me not to, but I'm just not as interested as I once was. Watch for changes like these and record them in your Journal.
- You may choose foods more for how they make you feel rather than how they taste. Your body will tell you what it needs to run smoothly and what drags it down. Part of the harmony with food is this

acceptance of food as an agent to get your whole self—body, mind *and* spirit—feeling better.

- You may want to experiment more with new foods. When you realize how good foods taste and how good they are for you, you will want to open yourself up to new experiences. I wasn't surprised when one of my meat-and-potatoes students started branching off into foods he'd never tried before. It comes with the CAMP territory.
- You may lose some interest in most beverages. After clearing for a number of weeks, I found myself virtually ignoring all other beverages. Water became my drink of choice and more and more important for the enjoyment of food, and other than my orange juice for breakfast or a cup of coffee in the morning, I rarely have any other liquid at my meals.
- It will seem as if your stomach is getting smaller and smaller. Even if you force yourself to eat the old way, you'll find that you can't anymore. And if you do eat beyond your capacity (the way you used to) you'll learn how uncomfortable and draining on the body's energy that is.
- You find yourself getting creative with your eating. One of my students came up with this strategy: when she orders at a restaurant, she tells the waiter to put half of her order in a take-home container even before he brings it to the table. She's less tempted to eat the food then, and she has dinner for another night. Another CAMPer uses the clock creatively. He times his meal, eating a normal meal for, say, 25 minutes—whenever he gets to the end of 25 minutes, he stops. If one week he see that he's gaining a little weight, he changes his meal time to 20 minutes of eating for each meal (thus eating less food). If he's losing more weight than he wants to, he eats for 30 minutes each meal (thus increasing his food intake). Let your creative juices flow as you customize the CAMP system for your own life.

Tuning In Deeper

In chapter 9 we examined the idea of tuning in to the body to find out what it wants and how it feels. It's important to do that, but it's only the surface. The CAMP system operates at three levels: body, mind and spirit.

All three are worthy of tuning in to, and with time and practice we can learn to do that.

When we tune in to the body, we learn about its nutritional needs, what foods support the body's functions and what foods get in the way.

When we tune in to the mind, we learn how food enhances our emotional life, our sensations and our psychological needs. And as we come into more and more control over food and defeat its power over us, we reach a harmony point were we know we are in command of food. It's no longer "food over mind," but rather "mind over food."

Finally, as we tune in to the spirit, whatever that means to us, we begin to see how food influences and supports what we're here on earth to do. We get closer to understanding the role food plays in getting us closer to our goals as human beings and how its misuse can get in the way of our noblest purposes. By embracing mindfulness while eating, we feed our own spirits with great richness and help them grow and develop.

That kind of harmony, that involves all three aspects of our personalities, is the most profound goal of the CAMP system, and can fill the rest of our lives with exciting exploration.

In Closing

The adventure in the CAMP system may appear to be over because you're nearly at the end of this book, but actually the adventure is just beginning. You have a lifetime of eating ahead.

There will be times when you'll slip back a little and there will be events in life that test you. Review this book often and do the practices again and again. Don't give up on your Journal: those five minutes every evening recording your eating are your anchor and will keep you on the mindful path.

Above all, with every meal and every encounter with food:

Relax. Arrive. Be attentive.

Enjoy. Taste. Feel. Smell. See.

Open up. Savor. Slow down. Take your time.

Be deliberate. Appreciate. Have fun.

Give thanks. Don't rush. Experience every bite.

Take only what you need. Be in harmony. Treat yourself well.

Be gracious. Live in dignity.

Practice: Chocolate!

Chocolate may not be the food of the gods, but it's a close second to whatever is. There's no need to deny ourselves an occasional self-indulgence, and chocolate is an excellent way to experience the full depth of extravagance in a controlled, CAMP-like way.

Chocolate's gifts are rich and profuse. It's full of energy, carbohydrates and fats. It's bursting with flavor and dark, creamy texture. We must honor it well by enjoying small encounters, during which we extract every moment of chocolate pleasure.

Select a piece of chocolate to enjoy. I prefer the individually wrapped, small chocolate candies that are easy to break into two pieces. These are usually square and wrapped in foil. (If you don't like chocolate, select a sweet treat that you do like.) You might select chocolate with peanuts, almonds or rice crisps in it, but I prefer the plain, pure, unadulterated milk chocolate for the authentic chocolate experience.

For this exercise, you'll need a single chocolate candy, some water for clearing, a watch or clock with a second hand and a few minutes quietly alone. For the next moments it will be just you and the chocolate and the perfection of its mindful consumption.

1. Before you open the wrapper, arrive at the chocolate. Consider the gift of this food. Chocolate is a product of the tropical cocoa plant. Materials from

the bean (or fruit) of this plant are mixed with milk, milk solids, and cocoa fat or other fats. Somewhere in Central or South America, workers had to gather and process the beans from the plant so that you could enjoy this candy today. Appreciate their efforts. Feel the chocolate in your hand. Smell the chocolate even through the wrapper. Begin your enjoyment of the chocolate now. If it has one, read the label on the wrapper and see exactly what's in the food.

2. Unwrap the chocolate slowly, carefully, thoughtfully. Enjoying chocolate is a sensuous experience and so is the expectation of eating it. Take your time with opening the candy, peeling back the layers of foil until the food is completely exposed.

3. Fresh chocolate has a wonderful aroma. Put your nose close to the chocolate, close your eyes and take three deep breaths. Linger in the depths of the sultry fragrance.

4. Break the chocolate in half. You're going to eat one half at a time, and you want to spend at least 90 seconds with each half. Take one of the halves and place it in your mouth. Notice where the second hand on the clock is. Don't chew the chocolate; rather, just let it sit on the tongue. Notice the feel of chocolate in your mouth and how it begins to change after 10 or 15 seconds. Let the warmth of your mouth warm the candy.

5. As the chocolate starts to melt, move it slowly across the tongue, allowing the chocolate to melt as a pat of butter melts on a warm skillet. Coat the entire inner surfaces of your mouth with creamy liquid chocolate. Feel its smoothness, richness and sweetness. Close your eyes to enhance the experience.

6. From time to time as the chocolate melts, allow yourself to swallow some of the melted candy. Follow it down your esophagus into your stomach.

7. Keep the chocolate in your mouth as long as you can, but at least for 90 seconds. When you have swallowed all the chocolate, stop.

8. Before clearing, notice the aftertastes. Swallow again and watch the changing tastes in your mouth. Smile that you have another half of chocolate to enjoy. Pause as you find yourself deep within this ultimate chocolate experience.

9. Clear with water, several times if necessary. You want to return your mouth to its previous pre-chocolate condition.

10. Enjoy the second piece of chocolate in the same way as the first. Imagine that this is your very first piece of chocolate ever—see it with fresh eyes and taste it with fresh mouth.

11. If part of the chocolate experience you enjoy is chewing it, allow yourself to chew up the remaining chocolate in your mouth near the end of the second 90 seconds. When it's thoroughly chewed, swallow.

12. After you swallow this second half, again pause.

13. Clear with water.

14. Smile that you've just enjoyed chocolate more than anyone on earth ever has. You don't need a bag of chocolate or even a handful; decide that one piece is quite enough.

Repeat this exercise several times each week. Develop your own style and rituals for enjoying this wonderful food.

And may every meal bring you joy, every bite bring you harmony, every taste bring you grace, every morsel bring you balance and peace.

16.

Frequently Asked Questions about the CAMP System

How do I know how much I should eat during a meal?

Learning how much to eat takes time and effort. You need to pay attention to your body, how you feel throughout the meal and for hours afterwards. Several times during each meal you should stop and take a moment to ask yourself if you're getting what you need. If not, keep eating. If so, stop. Sometimes, you may even stop while you're still a little hungry, because you know that as you continue to digest your food the hunger will go away.

As a CAMPer, can I have snacks?

By all means. Remember, what's important is not what you eat, but rather how you eat it. If you feel you need a snack, go ahead and enjoy. Eat the snack as you would any food: slowly, carefully, attentively and mindfully. Make your bites small. Between each bite, clear with water. If you're going to have a flavored beverage with your snack, treat it as a food—after each sip, clear with water. Honor the snack by taking only what you need and no more. The snack you eat is another great gift of food, and you want to show it the utmost respect.

Having said all that, I have to remind you: *snacking is perhaps the number one form of overeating.* To stop or limit snacks is one of the best ways to control weight. If you must snack, do so as I've outlined above, but if you can eliminate or reduce your snacking comfortably, even better.

The hardest thing about the CAMP system is remembering to do it. I'll find myself eating away at a meal only to realize that I should have been doing the CAMP system but forgot. How do I remember to do it?

Remembering to eat in the CAMP way is difficult, especially for new CAMPers. The key is how you arrive at food. To "arrive" means that you're aware that food has come into your life and that you have tasks to do. Here are a few strategies. When you first sit down to a meal, take four deep breaths. Or perhaps say to yourself, "Wake up!" At home, ring a small bell at the beginning of each meal. Sit quietly until the sound completely fades away. The idea here is to develop habits of becoming aware of your food. Later on, as the habit takes hold, you will automatically remember to do the system.

I have too many distractions when I eat. How do I keep my mind on the system?

You have to ask yourself just how important is it to get into balance and harmony with food. If you find yourself being distracted, *it's only because you are allowing yourself to be distracted.* If you decide to make the CAMP system one of the most important things in your life, you will. The other factors competing for your attention will not have the power they did any more. If you find yourself distracted, ask yourself why you're allowing yourself to be pulled away from the system. The answer will reveal much about where you're placing your priorities.

Is it okay to just have a regular meal once in a while, without all the steps and rules?

Follow your heart. If friends ask me to go out for hard-shelled crabs and beer, I will probably say yes. I know that I'll likely eat more than I should and not clear with water and perhaps have a little more beer than I should. But I know that it's for a special occasion and is not the normal type of meal I eat. I still can eat the crabs mindfully.

Recently, my wife and I went to a five-course wine dinner for Valentine's Day. Every course had a sparkling wine, and the menu included oysters, shrimp, duck and (of all things) venison. Although the servings were somewhat small, it was still a huge meal by my standards. I ate this meal in a CAMP way, taking my time and enjoying it fully. Did I eat more than I should? Yes, but I knew it was a very special meal and I was aware to honor the food even though I took a little extra.

The CAMP system was never meant to be a rigid series of rules and regulations. Rather, it is a way of redirecting the mind to see food in a new way, to experience eating in a natural and balanced way. If you feel the need to abandon those ideas for a meal occasionally, that's fine, but my guess is that the longer you're on the CAMP system the more you'll see it as a way of life rather than as a set of rules to follow.

Can't I clear with iced tea? Water doesn't do much for me.

Clearing is very important to the CAMP system—it sets up your taste buds for the next bite, tricking the mouth into thinking the each bite is the first. Water is neutral, without flavor or aroma, and serves to clear the palate perfectly. Stop thinking of water as a beverage and see it in its new role. If you still want iced tea, include it in your meals. Just remember to treat the tea as a food.

Can I be on the CAMP system and a diet at the same time?

Yes. Remember, however, that many diets place restrictions on the types of foods you eat. These restrictions can lead to feelings of being deprived, and that goes against the first and most important of the CAMP principles: Never feel deprived.

If you wish to stay on your diet, though, that's your choice. You will likely find that eating your diets foods under the CAMP system makes them more enjoyable and satisfying. You'll be spending more time with your food, and the clearing between bites can make the food even more appetizing.

When do I go off of the CAMP system?

The CAMP system is a new way of eating based on a change of attitudes and arriving at balance and harmony with food. As such, it is a permanent method of eating.

I'm having trouble eating with the CAMP system at business meetings and parties. There's simply too much going on for me to keep it all straight. What can I do?

Parties, business lunches, holiday meals and other times can be difficult, but over time you can train yourself to maintain the CAMP system even in these situations. The key is in reminding yourself *every time you encounter food* that you have a lot of work to do. You must arrive at the food. Try four deep breaths. Try shouting (to yourself, of course), "Wake up! Food is here! I can't treat this lightly! I have steps to follow! Wake up!" Try imagining that any bit of food you have is like nitroglycerine: very dangerous if mishandled. You can't afford to take food for granted anymore.

If you practice these techniques bite by bite, meal by meal, day by day, you'll get in the habit of seeing food as very special but quite hazardous if not used correctly. Later, at the business lunch or the cocktail party, the sight and smell of food will trigger the same response. You'll go on your guard. You'll treat food as special and with all the great respect it deserves. And all of this can be going on while you're doing business or enjoying the conversation! (No one has to know.)

Since I'm supposed to be eating less, wouldn't it just be easier to skip meals? If I don't eat lunch every day, don't I get the benefit of not taking in all those calories?

On the surface it seems to make sense to skip meals, but oddly enough you can actually *gain* weight by skipping meals. Here's how it works: when you skip a meal, your body thinks that maybe food is getting scarce. To protect itself and to get the most of the food it gets, your body puts your metabolism on the 'slow' setting. As you skip more and more meals, this setting becomes the normal for you. Then, later, when you decide to have lunch again, the body receives a lot of extra food. But wait—your metabolic rate is on simmer. So all that extra food gets converted to fat, and you gain weight.

Instead of skipping meals, you should consider having more (but smaller) meals throughout the day. This is easiest on your digestive system and keeps your metabolism working at a much higher level.

I'm not doing very well with the CAMP Journal. Couldn't I just skip doing the Journal?

You could, but you shouldn't. The Journal has many long-term benefits (review the chapter on the Journal if you've forgotten them). I've had students who have told me they don't like doing the Journal or that they simply stopped writing. I then ask them they are losing weight or feeling more in balance with food, and every time I hear that they aren't having much success. The CAMP Journal is an important part of the system. But more importantly, if you find yourself looking for some reason to stop writing in your Journal, you should ask yourself what's going on. It's a great time to evaluate how important food control *really is* in your life. You may be surprised by your answer.

*The CAMP system asks me to slow down my eating, but I don't
have the time to eat so slowly. My life is so hectic that I have to
eat on the run and try to get my meals down as fast as
possible. What do I do?*

Eating on the run is not so terrible and trying to get meals down
quickly can be okay. The problem comes in when you get out of
balance with food and you misuse it, don't honor it and give it less
attention than it deserves. All too often the result of this
mistreatment of food is weight gain, which may be why you're
reading this book right now.

You have some important choices to make. Look at your schedule
and the way you fit into it. Look at your life and where you're
putting your attention. What is really important to you? I'd guess
that very few people would ask to have put on their tombstones, "I
wish I had rushed around more in my life." Sadly, many more
could use the epitaph "I should have lost weight sooner."

If controlling your weight is high on your priority list, then you
have to reorganize to accommodate that stance. You have to make
more time for yourself and how you treat food. *Find the time.* If
it's important enough for you, you will do it. And if you feel like
you're a prisoner of your hectic schedule, you may be out of
balance in more ways than you suspect.

*Friends or family members don't seem to like my new way of
eating. I get comments like, "Don't take so much time with
your food," or "Eat up, now, I'm finished." How do I handle
comments or even hostility from others?*

This is a tough one, often made more difficult because others may
actually resent your ability to eat less and enjoy it more than they
do. Keep in mind that at the very center of this issue is the concept
of control. Who will you let control your eating? If you find
yourself thinking, "I could eat less food more mindfully, but I have
to hurry up for my spouse/parent/friend/," you are really giving up
your power to your spouse or parent or friend.

155

I recommend that you talk to the people with whom you'll be eating. Tell them a little about what you'll be doing and why it's important to you. Let them know how they can support you and hope for their cooperation. But in the end, it's up to you to keep your power. Eat for *you*, not for others. And consider this: when others make remarks about how you are eating, they're really not commenting on you. Rather, they are making statements about themselves and their own problems and desires with food. Understand what they're saying, and don't take their comments personally.

Some foods, like ice cream or cereal with milk, require that you eat them rather quickly (otherwise, they melt or get soggy). How do you eat these foods slowly, in the CAMP way?

By changing portions, if you can. If you want a bowl of ice cream, get half a bowl and eat it slowly. Then, get some more (but only if you think you *really* need it!) The same would be true for cereal. Pour half a bowl and some milk. Eat it slowly, putting your spoon down between each bite and clearing with water after each bite. Then take some more cereal and milk, but only if you need it.

I'm finding myself getting obsessed with the CAMP system. My meals are getting smaller and smaller and whenever I ask myself if I really need more food I answer 'no' even though I probably do. This can't be healthy, can it?

No. The CAMP system is about balance and harmony, not about obsessing. You should be feeling good about your eating, regardless of how much. Concern yourself more with the techniques of eating—slowing down, chewing thoroughly, enjoying the food, clearing with water, eating mindfully—rather than with the quantity of food. If you eat with purpose and attention, gradually the food portions will take care of themselves. Also, take another look at the Food Economy on page 37 and remember that it's just as dangerous to spend too much time in *either* diagram A or C.

About the Author

Fred Burggraf is a native son of Indiana, Pennsylvania, where he attended undergraduate school at Indiana University of Pennsylvania.

During his career, Fred has taught high school science and has worked in the private sector as a business writer and editor, graphics specialist and communication specialist. In 1983, he received a Master's of Education degree from the University of Maryland.

Since 1992, Fred has worked as a consultant with smoking-cessation groups, helping people quit through a program similar to the CAMP system.

Fred is the author of *Thinking Connections: Concept Maps for Life Science* (published by Critical Thinking Books and Software) and his self-published *Quit Smoking for Good: A Workbook for Success in Smoking Cessation*.

Fred lives with his wife and their two dogs in Southern Maryland. He enjoys birding, classical music, antiques, composing hymns, completing crossword puzzles and, of course, eating well.

Learn more about the CAMP system at **www.MindfulEating.net**
www.MindfulEating.org